D0505983

HEALTH IMPACTS OF LARGE RELEASES OF RADIONUCLIDES

The Ciba Foundation is an international scientific and educational charity (Registered Charity No. 313574). It was established in 1947 by the Swiss chemical and pharmaceutical company of CIBA Limited — now Ciba-Geigy Limited. The Foundation operates independently in London under English trust law.

The Ciba Foundation exists to promote international cooperation in biological, medical and chemical research. It organizes about eight international multidisciplinary symposia each year on topics that seem ready for discussion by a small group of research workers. The papers and discussions are published in the Ciba Foundation symposium series. The Foundation also holds many shorter meetings (not published), organized by the Foundation itself or by outside scientific organizations. The staff always welcome suggestions for future meetings.

The Foundation's house at 41 Portland Place, London W1N 4BN, provides facilities for meetings of all kinds. Its Media Resource Service supplies information to journalists on all scientific and technological topics. The library, open five days a week to any graduate in science or medicine, also provides information on scientific meetings throughout the world and answers general enquiries on biomedical and chemical subjects. Scientists from any part of the world may stay in the house during working visits to London.

The European Environmental Research Organisation (EERO) was established in 1987 by a group of scientists from seven European countries. The members, now drawn from 14 countries, are scientists elected in recognition of their outstanding contributions to environmental research or training. EERO became fully operational in 1990 as a non-profit making, non-political foundation, with its offices at the Agricultural University of Wageningen, Generaal Foulkesweg 70, 6703 BW Wageningen, The Netherlands. EERO seeks to strengthen environmental research and training in Europe and neighbouring countries, from the Atlantic to the Urals, and from Scandinavia to the Mediterranean. It does so by promoting the most effective use of intellectual and technological resources and by supporting new and emerging scientific opportunities. EERO also provides a resource for authoritative but independent scientific assessment of environmental issues and institutions. Particular objectives are: to develop the potential of promising younger scientists by providing opportunities for collaborative research and training; to bring together participants from the relevant basic sciences to form interdisciplinary environmental research groups; to catalyse the formation and evolution of international networks to exploit emerging opportunities in environmental research; to facilitate the rapid spread in Europe of new theoretical knowledge from all parts of the world; to provide training in new developments in environmental science for those in government, industry and the research community; and to make independent scientific assessments of environmental problems and institutions, as a basis for advice to government or industry.

Ciba Foundation Symposium 203

HEALTH IMPACTS OF LARGE RELEASES OF RADIONUCLIDES

1997

JOHN WILEY & SONS

Chichester · New York · Weinheim · Brisbane · Singapore · Toronto

Published in 1997 by John Wiley & Sons Ltd,
Baffins Lane, Chichester,
West Sussex PO19 1UD, England

National 01243 779777
International (+44) 1243 779777
e-mail (for orders and customer service enquiries): cs-books@wiley.co.uk
Visit our Home Page on http://www.wiley.co.uk
or http://www.wiley.com

Other Wiley Editorial Offices

John Wiley & Sons, Inc., 605 Third Avenue,
New York, NY 10158-0012, USA

VCH Verlagsgesellschaft MbH, Pappelallee 3,
D-69469 Weinheim, Germany

Jacaranda Wiley Ltd, 33 Park Road, Milton,
Queensland 4064, Australia

John Wiley & Sons (Asia) Pte Ltd, 2 Clementi Loop #02-01,
Jin Xing Distripark, Singapore 0512

John Wiley & Sons (Canada) Ltd, 22 Worcester Road,
Rexdale, Ontario M9W 1L1, Canada

Ciba Foundation Symposium 203
x+247 pages, 37 figures, 30 tables

Library of Congress Cataloging-in-Publication Data

Health impacts of large releases of radionuclides.
　　　p.　cm. — (Ciba Foundation symposium ; 203)
　　　Editors: John V. Lake, Gregory R. Bock (organizers), and Gail Cardew.
　　　Includes bibliographical references and index.
　　　ISBN 0-471-96510-3 (alk. paper)
　　　1. Radioactive pollution — Health aspects — Congresses
　　2. Radioecology — Congresses.　3. Radioactive pollution —
　　Environmental aspects — Congresses.　I. Lake, J. V.　II. Bock,
　　Gregory.　III. Cardew, Gail.　IV. Series.
　　　[DNLM: 1. Radioisotopes — adverse effects — congresses.
　　2. Radiation Effects — congresses.　W3 C161F v. 203 1997 / WN 610
　　H4345 1997]
　　RA569.H378　1997
　　363.17'99 — dc21
　　DNLM/DLC
　　for Library of Congress　　　　　　　　　　　　　　97-294
　　　　　　　　　　　　　　　　　　　　　　　　　　　　　　CIP

British Library Cataloguing in Publication Data

A catalogue record for this book is available from the British Library

ISBN 0 471 96510 3

Typeset in 10/12pt Garamond by Dobbie Typesetting Limited, Tavistock, Devon.
Printed and bound in Great Britain by Biddles Ltd, Guildford.
This book is printed on acid-free paper responsibly manufactured from sustainable forestation, for which at least two trees are planted for each one used for paper production.

Contents

Participants

A. Aarkrog   Environmental Science and Technology Department MIL-114, Risø National Laboratory, PO Box 49, DK-4000 Roskilde, Denmark

M. I. Balonov   Radioecology Department, Institute of Radiation Hygiene, Mira Street 8, 197101 St Petersburg, Russia

M. Bauchinger   Institut für Strahlenbiologie, GSF-Forschungszentrum für Umwelt und Gesundheit, Postfach 1129, D-85758, Oberschleissheim, Germany

A. Blinov   Department of Cosmic Research, St Petersburg Technical University, Polytechnicheskaya 29, RO-195251 St Petersburg, Russia

A. A. Cigna   Fraz. Tuffo, I-14023 Cocconato AT, Italy

M. Frissel   Torenlaan 3, NL-6866- BS Heelsum, The Netherlands

G. M. Gadd   Department of Biological Sciences, University of Dundee, Dundee, DD1 4HN, UK

M. Goldman   Department of Radiological Sciences, University of California, 1122 Pine Lane, Davis, CA 95616–1729, USA

L. Håkanson   Institute of Earth Sciences, Uppsala University, Norbyvägen 18B, S-75236 Uppsala, Sweden

B. J. Howard   Institute of Terrestrial Ecology, Merlewood Research Station, Grange-over-Sands, Cumbria LA11 6JU, UK

A. Konoplev   Institute of Experimental Meteorology SPA 'Typhoon', Lenin av 82, Obninsk 249020, Russia

J. V. Lake   European Environmental Research Organisation, Generaal Foulkesweg 70, PO Box 191, NL-6700 AD Wageningen, The Netherlands

H. G. Paretzke   (*Chairman*) GSF, Institut für Strahlenschutz, Ingolstädter Landstrasse 1, 85764 Neuherberg, Germany

A. Prisyazhniuk   Scientific Centre for Radiation Medicine, Kiev, Ukraine

O. Renn   Center of Technology Assessment, Industriestrasse 5, D-70565 Stuttgart, Germany

J. Roed   Contamination Physics Group, Environmental Science and Technology Department, Risø National Laboratory, PO Box 49, DK-4000 Roskilde, Denmark

C. Streffer   Universitätsklinikum Essen, Institut für Medizinische Strahlenbiologie, Hufelandstrasse 55, D-45122 Essen, Germany

G. Voigt   GSF, Institut für Strahlenschutz, Ingolstädter Landstrasse 1, 85764 Neuherberg, Germany

F. W. Whicker   Department of Radiological Health Sciences, Colorado State University, Fort Collins, CO 80523, USA

Introduction

H. G. Paretzke

GSF, Institut für Strahlenschutz, Ingolstädter Landstrasse 1, 85764 Neuherberg, Germany

The potential health impacts of large releases of radionuclides have been of increasing interest during the last 50 years or so. This interest began with the atmospheric testing of nuclear bombs and continued with the use of nuclear energy. In the 1970s it was discovered that large amounts of radionuclides are released by other processes — for example, during volcanic eruptions — and there can also be a high level of radionuclides in waste rocks at the surface of silver and other mines.

Ten years after the catastrophic release of large amounts of radionuclides from the core material of the nuclear reactor at Chernobyl into the atmosphere and into aquatic environments, the Ciba Foundation and The European Environmental Research Organisation considered it appropriate to bring together a group of experts in the interdisciplinary fields of radiation protection, radiation research, environmental research and health research, so that the scientific knowledge obtained over the last 10 years could be discussed. During this symposium it will be possible to consider progress in our understanding of the transport of radionuclides in the environment, including the natural environment (which has largely been neglected by western radioecologists), the semi-natural environment, agricultural areas, the aquatic environment and urban areas. We will also discuss recent experiences on the various exposure pathways of radionuclides to humans.

It is only a few years ago that scientists first evaluated the scientific basis for the well-known statement made 30 years ago by the International Commission on Radiological Protection that if you protect human individuals against exposure to ionizing radiation, then the environment (i.e. both animal and plant populations) is also protected. This statement has not been checked experimentally in great detail, so we will also discuss this topic.

Often in this field we have to deal with the situation in which an individual's dose cannot be measured at the time of exposure and it therefore has to be estimated retrospectively. We will discuss this problem and solutions, as well as the negative effect on human health of such exposures. Finally, we will also learn about scientific approaches to evaluate the various psychological impacts of exposures to large releases of radionuclides.

When discussing the present state of our understanding in this complex field, we should focus on important, general aspects rather than on the nitty-gritty details. If we adopt such an approach we may be able to solve many general problems and lay down pathways for future research on the health and environmental impacts of large releases of radionuclides.

Physical transport and chemical and biological processes in agricultural systems

Gabriele Voigt

GSF, Institut für Strahlenschutz, Ingolstädter Landstrasse 1, 85764 Neuherberg, Germany

Abstract. The purpose of radioecological models is to make realistic estimates of doses to the public after accidental releases of radionuclides into the environment. Important physical, chemical and biological processes involved in the dispersion and transport of radioactive substances in the atmosphere and along the food-chains are presented. The results of the EURAD (EURopean Acid Deposition) model, predicting the deposition patterns of ^{131}I and ^{137}Cs in Belarus and Ukraine after the Chernobyl accident, are discussed. An overview of the most important ecological processes — such as deposition, interception and translocation, weathering, transfers from soil to plants and from plants to animal/animal products, and seasonality in agricultural environments — is given. Examples corresponding to these individual processes, mainly experimental results after the Chernobyl accident and related to radiocaesium and radioiodine, are shown and discussed.

1997 Health impacts of large releases of radionuclides. Wiley, Chichester (Ciba Foundation Symposium 203) p 3–20

It is important to assess the radiological consequences of accidental releases of radionuclides into the atmosphere and the resulting contamination of large areas. Rapid and detailed prognoses of the resulting radiation exposure to population groups are required in order to support and optimize decisions concerning countermeasures to keep doses as low as possible. Exposure pathways of importance are: (1) internal exposure due to the ingestion of contaminated foodstuffs and the inhalation of radionuclides during the passing of clouds; and (2) external exposure from radionuclides during the passing of clouds, and the deposition of radionuclides on the ground and other surfaces.

One of the major exposure pathways, especially in the short- and medium-term after an accident, results from the deposition of radionuclides on agriculturally cultivated land used for the production of plant and animal foodstuffs for human nutrition. For estimating the internal dose due to ingestion, information on the different dynamic processes leading to the time-dependent contamination of food (such as the transport

3

of radionuclides in the atmosphere, their deposition on vegetation and their transfer through the food-chains) is required. These processes are influenced by many factors, such as the conditions during the release (e.g. temperature of the reactor, and height and physical composition of the source), the meteorological conditions and season during dispersion and fallout, the type of deposition, and the physico-chemical form of the radionuclide. Information on these processes is available in agricultural systems where realistic data could be obtained after the Chernobyl accident. These different processes are discussed here, and the corresponding results obtained mainly after the Chernobyl accident are also presented.

Atmospheric dispersion

Following nuclear accidents or incidents, radioactivity is released into the lower layers of the atmosphere and can then be transported into higher air layers by thermal lift, resulting in a distribution according to the meteorological conditions. Different physical and chemical processes have to be considered in order to estimate the degree of contamination of different areas. These include: the spatial and temporal changes in meteorological conditions (such as wind speed, temperature, turbulence, pressure, three-dimensional advection, and vertical and horizontal diffusion); transformation or decay processes; deposition conditions and precipitation; the structure of surfaces; and landuse.

After the Chernobyl accident radioactive material was found all over the Northern hemisphere. Long-range transport resulted in a substantial contamination (after one week) of areas thousands of kilometres away from the Chernobyl nuclear plant (e.g. Finland, the Alps and Greece). This demonstrates that the movement of plumes deriving from such accidents can be complex. Different models describing the spatial and temporal distribution of radioactivity are based on observed meteorological fields. These include trajectory calculations, Lagrangian models (Apsimon & Wilson 1987, Albergel et al 1988) and Eulerian models (Pudykiewicz 1988, Gudiksen et al 1989). For verification, the calculated activity concentrations using these models have been compared with radiological measurements in air, water and soil samples. Most of these comparisons were in relatively good agreement.

Some of the major sources of uncertainty in modelling and reconstructing the dispersion after an accident are the quantifications of the source term, and the physical and chemical conditions at the reactor during the release. In particular, information that describes the time-dependent variation of the radionuclide composition, the temperature and the effective release height is required. In the case of the Chernobyl accident, models such as PATRIC, a three-dimensional sequential

---

FIG. 1.   (*opposite*) Correlations between the measured and estimated dry (A) and wet (B) ^{137}Cs soil depositions in 4500 settlements in northern Ukraine (using the EURopean Acid Deposition [EURAD] model).

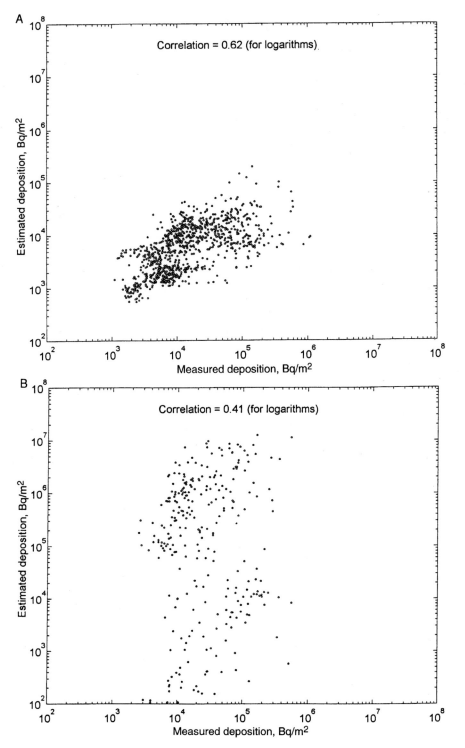

transport and diffusion model for long-range effects (Lange et al 1988) or MESO/ REGION for short-range effects (Borzilov & Klepikova 1993) have estimated the source term. These estimates are likely to be within a factor of two to three of the actual amount released, calculated on the basis of radionuclide inventories and direct measurements above and in the vicinity of the reactor (Buzulukov & Dobrynin 1993). The main release height was estimated to be about 1700 m. This was determined by vertical profiles, and therefore it is assumed that most of the long-range dispersion of radioactivity occurred at about 1500 m (GRS 1987).

In contrast to the models mentioned above, the EURAD (EURopean Acid Deposition) model (Hass et al 1990) uses predictive meteorological fields and assesses the Eulerian model system EURAD in a forecast mode. By keeping the assumptions, parameters and source estimation as simple as possible, this model can be used flexibly to simulate the situation in both a predictive and retrospective way. The model was compared with measured air activity data for several European areas and was in reasonably good agreement with the observations, thus validating the predictive capacity in emergency situations. We applied the EURAD model to reconstruct short-range ^{131}I deposition after the Chernobyl accident, i.e. in northern Ukraine and southern Belarus, in a 10 km grid in order to reconstruct thyroid doses to children (G. Voigt, H. Geiss and H. G. Paretzke, unpublished results 1995). We tested the reliability of the model's predictions together with colleagues in the Belorussian Institute of Radiation Medicine in Belarus and the Lawrence Livermore Laboratory in the USA by comparing the ^{137}Cs activities calculated by the EURAD model with direct measurements made by official Ukrainian Authorities. Figure 1 shows that contamination derived from dry deposition is relatively well determined, whereas that from wet deposition requires further evaluation. The discrepancy is mainly due to the high artificial precipitation rates assumed in the meteorological model and a movement prediction of the plume that was too fast.

Deposition

Two fallout processes of radionuclides on agricultural land can be distinguished, i.e. dry and wet deposition.

Dry deposition

This relates to the deposition of particles or gaseous substances on underground soil or plant surfaces near the soil surface. The process itself is rather complex and can be described by three individual steps: the aerodynamic resistance; the surface layer resistance; and the transfer resistance. The aerodynamic resistance represents the transport from the free atmosphere to the laminar boundary surface layer. It is influenced by meteorological factors, such as wind speed and turbulence, and also by the structure of the surface in question. Data are available (Hosker & Lindberg 1982) comparing the relative aerodynamic resistance in different plant canopies. For example, after dry deposition in pastures the relative aerodynamic resistance can be up to 50%,

TABLE 1 Deposition velocities for ^{137}Cs aerosols and gaseous ^{131}I on pasture grass after the Chernobyl accident

Radioisotope	Deposition velocity (mm/s)	Yield (g/m³ dry matter)	Reference
^{137}Cs	0.30–1.5	0.10	Bonka et al 1986
	0.17–0.44	0.04	Roed 1987
	0.63–0.87	0.17	Roed 1987
^{131}I	5.00–10.0	0.15–0.2	Bonka et al 1986
	1.80–12.0	0.04–0.19	Roed 1987

depending on the grass density, whereas in forests this figure can be as low as 10%. Therefore, the deposition of material is more effective on more developed plant canopies, and a linear relationship between leaf area index and the amount of deposition can be assumed (Wedding et al 1975). The surface layer resistance can be described by diffusion, impaction and sedimentation, according to both the size of the particles or material and the structure and condition of the surface itself. Transfer resistances involve the interaction between the deposited material and the surface layer. This process involves chemical and physical interactions, depending on valency, loading and size of the ion.

These parameters determine the extent of the transfer into biological material. They are partly independent, but are difficult to separate. Therefore, the amount of deposited material is expressed by the deposition velocity and the concentration in the air near the ground. The deposition velocity can be measured, but only limited experimental data are currently available. It is possible that more information will be obtained in the light of the Chernobyl accident. The deposition velocity is strongly correlated with the size of the leaf surface and the aerosol diameter. For example, in Germany and Austria about 80% of the ^{137}Cs activity was bound to 0.1–1.0 μm aerosols (Tschiersch & Georgii 1987), and deposition velocities of 0.3–1.5 mm/s were reported on pasture grass, depending on the yield (Roed 1987, Bonka et al 1986, Table 1). For iodine the situation is more complicated because of the different chemical forms that behave differently during deposition. Iodine in its elementary form (as iodine gas) deposits 10-fold faster than aerosol-bound iodine, and iodine bound to organic matter deposits 10-fold more slowly than aerosol-bound iodine. Long-range (>100 km from the source) assumed deposition rates in fully developed pastures are: 1.5 mm/s for aerosol-bound iodine; 15 mm/s for iodine gas; and 0.15 mm/s for iodine organically bound or in organic form.

Within the dynamic radioecological model, ECOSYS, describing the transfer of radionuclides through food-chains (Müller & Pröhl 1993), the total dry deposition on plant and soil is represented by:

$$D_d(T) = D_p(T) + D_s(T) = v_p(T) + v_s c_a.$$

Where $D_d(T)$ = total dry deposition (Bq/m^2); $D_p(T)$ = dry deposition on plants (Bq/m^2); $D_s(T)$ = dry deposition on soil (Bq/m^2); $v_p(T)$ deposition velocity for plants (m/s); v_s = deposition velocity for soil (m/s); and c_a = time-integrated air concentration in ground near air ($Bq \, s/m^3$).

The assumptions made in this model are in agreement with measurements made after the Chernobyl accident, which are well documented in the national and international literature.

Wet deposition

Wet deposition of radionuclides occurs with precipitation of rain, snow or fog. Only the processes concerned with rainfall are considered in this chapter. The fraction retained by plants is represented by the interception factor. It depends upon the water storage capacity of the plants (for pasture grass a mean value of 0.23 mm is reasonable), which may change according to the plant's developmental stage, the plant species and its morphological characteristics, and the chemical and physical form of the deposited radionuclide (e.g. values for iodine are twofold lower than for caesium, and those for strontium are twofold higher than for caesium). The fraction of rain retained by a plant is therefore dependent on the radionuclide, the water storage capacity, the leaf area index and the amount of rain (Fig. 2).

The level of contamination in plants after wet and dry deposition is attributable to the developmental stage of the plants. During the growing season the plant's morphology changes markedly, and this influences the interception of both dry and wet deposition. Therefore, the season during which the fallout occurs has a major impact on the extent of contamination because of differences in both climatic conditions and the developmental stage of the plant.

Biological transport processes

Once radionuclides have been deposited onto leaves, radioactive ions can be transferred via the epidermis and the cuticle into the inner plant parts, and gaseous compounds are taken up via the stomata into the plant. Both processes depend, for example, on the plant species, the nutritional state of the plant and the relative humidity in the surrounding air. For the contamination of plants, and especially edible plant parts, shortly after fallout, weathering and translocation after leaf uptake are important.

Weathering

Radionuclides deposited on plants are subject to weathering. Three processes can be distinguished: wash-off of adherent radionuclides; wash-out (leaching) of already absorbed radionuclides; and senescence. These losses are influenced by many factors, such as chemical parameters, vegetation, growth rate, soil resuspension, wind removal and run-off from leaves. Results of experiments obtained for *Lolium perenne* after a single

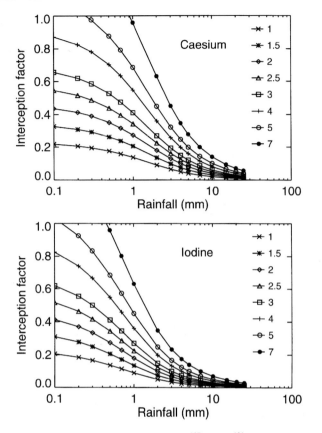

FIG. 2. Dependence of the interception factors for ^{137}Cs and ^{131}I on the amount of rain and the leaf area index (represented by different symbols).

contamination at GSF Institut für Strahlenschutz indicate that at least two different processes can be quantified experimentally. These processes are reflected by two effective half-lives with values of three days (90%) for an initial rapid removal and 23 days (10%) for a slow decrease (related to dry weight) (Fig. 3, Ertel et al 1989). After the Chernobyl accident, the mean effective weathering half-life for radiocaesium was estimated at the GSF Institut für Strahlenschutz as 20–25 days, taking into account growth dilution. This is in accordance with data in the literature (ISS 1986, Müller & Pröhl 1988).

Transport within the plant/translocation

Transport of an absorbed radionuclide within the plant generally depends on its mobility. Therefore, mobile and immobile elements can be distinguished. Alkaline

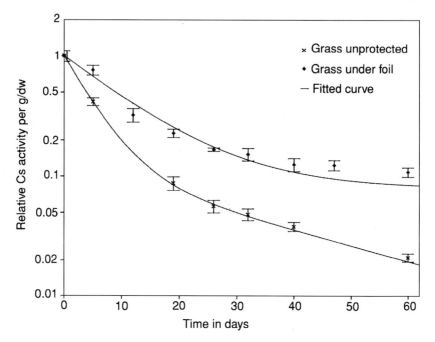

FIG. 3.   Weathering of ^{137}Cs on *Lolium perenne* after single-leaf contamination.

metals and iodine are highly mobile and are transported within the phloem (assimilation stream in both directions) and the xylem (transpiration stream from root to leaf). In contrast, strontium, for example, is practically immobile because it reacts with phosphate, resulting in the build-up of insoluble salts that are retained in the phloem. When radionuclides are taken up via foliage, translocation from leaves into the different plant organs takes place. This process is described by the translocation factor—defined as the fraction of total activity deposited on the plant in relation to the activity found in the edible plant parts, which can reach values of up to 10–15%. For example, the relationship between the translocation factor and the time before harvest is shown in Fig. 4 for ^{137}Cs in grain exposed to rain water from Chernobyl after the accident (Voigt et al 1991). This also demonstrates the strong seasonal dependency of the process.

The main factors affecting contamination are, therefore, the activity initially deposited on the leaves, the time between deposition and harvest, the yield, and the translocation factor to the edible part of the plant. Contamination by leaf uptake is maximum when the accident occurs while the green parts of vegetation (early in the season) or the edible parts (shortly before harvest) are exposed. However, the process of resuspension also has to be taken into account. In highly contaminated regions, such as in the 30 km zone around Chernobyl, resuspension can contribute significantly to

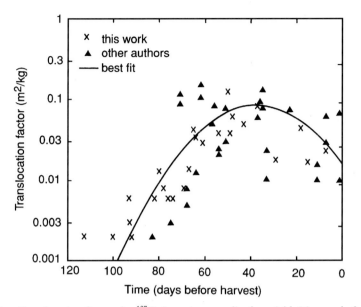

FIG. 4.   Translocation factors for ^{137}Cs in grain normalized to yield. Measured after a single contamination event at different stages in plant development. Other authors are Aarkrog (1969, 1972) and Middleton (1959).

the contamination of vegetation and the inhalation doses (Garger et al 1996). With respect to the long-term effects, however, transfer via root uptake and subsequent transport will dominate the fluxes within plants.

Root uptake

Transfer via root uptake is a complicated process that is influenced by many factors. For quantification, the transfer factor is expressed as the fraction of the activity concentrated in the plant (fresh weight) in relation to the activity concentrated in the zone near the root (dry weight). There is also a strong correlation between caesium and potassium uptake in soils with a low potassium content (because of the similarities between caesium and potassium). The root uptake of caesium is dependent on the clay and humus content, as well as the pH, of the soil. Therefore, transfer factors reported in the literature generally show a high level of variation; for example, transfer factors for pasture grass of 0.001–0.08 have been reported. Almost all the reported transfer factors determined before and after the Chernobyl accident for different plant species have been collected and evaluated by the International Union of Radioecologists (IUR) group working on soil to plant transfer factors (see Frissel 1992). Transfer factors for radiocaesium can be dramatically higher on agricultural land that is used extensively (semi-natural and natural ecosystems) and in soils with a low nutritional state. On land used for agriculture, transfer factors of 0.05 for pasture grass, and 0.02 for grain and vegetables are used in the ECOSYS model (Müller & Pröhl 1993), which are reasonable values for European conditions with well-fertilized soils.

A close relationship exists between root uptake and the leaching of radionuclides from the soil zone near the root into the deeper soil layers where they are not available for plant uptake. Leaching is due to water infiltration and migration by chemical and biological processes. The migration rate can change in the different soil horizons depending on the soil characteristics (moisture, clay content, soil density and organic substances) and the water infiltration velocity. [137]Cs migration rates have been determined for a German grassland soil. These are about 1–2 cm/y for the Chernobyl fallout and 0.3–1 cm/y for weapons fallout (K. Bunzl, personal communication 1996). The resistance time of a radionuclide in the soil layers can also be expressed by the K_d (partition coefficient) value, which is defined as the activity absorbed per unit soil related to the soluble activity in the soil solution. For caesium, the K_d value is about 1000 cm^3/g, and for strontium about 100 cm^3/g (Bachhuber et al 1984). However, the leaching process is only of minor importance for radiocaesium, due to its rapid fixation in the soil and slow migration rates.

Transfer to animals

The feeding of contaminated fodder to animals results in the contamination of animals and animal products consumed by humans. Meat and milk are the main contributors to human ingestion doses, especially in the first year after an accident. The transfer of fodder to milk or meat is usually described by the transfer coefficient, which gives the ratio of activity in one kilogram of meat or milk to the daily activity intake, assuming equilibrium conditions. After the Chernobyl accident, transfer coefficients were experimentally determined at the GSF Institut für Strahlenschutz for the products of different animal species relevant for human nutrition in Germany (Voigt et al 1989a,b, 1993a). A summary of these results for ^{137}Cs is given in Table 2. For ^{131}I milk transfer coefficients have been estimated as 0.0015–0.0081 kg/day (see Voigt et al 1989a).

The large variations in radionuclide transfer coefficients can be attributed to animal variables (such as breed, physiology, age and lactation stage) and dietary variables (such as vegetation species, feed combinations, diet selection and soil ingestion). Some of these factors influencing caesium, iodine and strontium transfer in ruminants have been subjected to the intensive investigations of a European research group and can be quantified (Voigt et al 1993b, EC 1995).

Subsequent to the Chernobyl accident, the behaviour of radiocaesium has been followed in a Bavarian farm (Voigt et al 1996). [137]Cs activity concentrated in milk from this farm is shown in Fig. 5. (The corresponding transfer coefficients for 1986–1995 are 0.0035, 0.004, 0.002, 0.007, 0.01, 0.0095, 0.01 and 0.009, for each respective year [Voigt et al 1996].) Transfer coefficients from feed to milk for radiocaesium

TABLE 2 Transfer coefficients and biological half-lives for ^{137}Cs after the Chernobyl accident for different animal products and reduction factors due to feed additives[a]

Animal product	Transfer coefficient (kg/day)	Half-life (days)	Bentonite	AFCF[b]
Cow's milk	0.0023–0.0053	1.5(0.8)–15(0.2)[c]	3.7	5.5
Beef (cow)	0.01	20–30	4.3	4.0
Beef (heifer)	0.035–0.04	50–60		
Beef (bull)	0.030–0.04	30–40		
Veal	0.035–0.40	25–30		
Pork	0.035–0.40	30–40	1.9	9.1
Sheep's milk	0.06			
Mutton	0.30–0.35	35–40		
Fallow deer meat	0.25–0.30	25–30		
Chicken (egg)	0.2/0.4[d]	2.8/3.2[d]		3/10
Chicken (breast)	1.6/3.0	25/15		4/8
Chicken (leg)	1.2/2.8	13/8		4/14

[a]Experiments not performed where values are missing.
[b]Ammonium ferrocyanoferrate (Giese salt, Prussian Blue).
[c]Figures in brackets represent the range.
[d]The first value refers to experiments performed with cobs feeding, and the second to wheat feeding.

originating from the Chernobyl accident have been determined by different groups (Ward & Johnson 1989, Solheim-Hansen & Hove 1991, Beresford et al 1992) and bioavailability has been reported to increase with time after deposition. We have confirmed that this increase occurred throughout the five years following the accident. The transfer of ^{137}Cs from soil to plant via root uptake has been described as identical for fallout resulting from weapons testing and the Chernobyl accident by Selnaes & Strand (1992). This implies that other mechanisms are involved in the contamination of pasture grass in the first three years after the accident (such as direct contamination, rain splash and resuspension); but that from 1989, root uptake of radiocaesium in a more bioavailable form was the predominant pathway.

Conclusion

The processes involved in determining the radionuclide fluxes via food-chains have been outlined here in a condensed form. The experimental data presented have been subjected to radioecological models created to provide or predict the expected dose to humans after radioactive contamination of large areas. It is important to understand these processes and to present both qualitative and quantitative data, so that effective countermeasures may be undertaken. Agricultural ecosystems have relatively well-

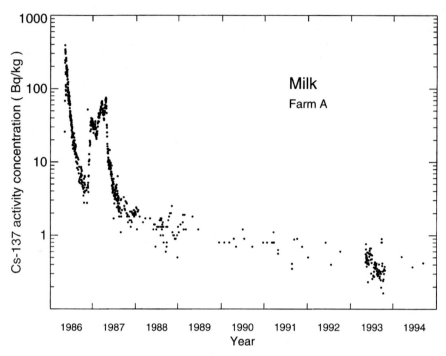

FIG. 5. [137]Cs activity concentration in milk from a Bavarian dairy farm measured at various times after the Chernobyl accident.

defined conditions, and therefore they have been used to study radionuclide fluxes following the Chernobyl accident. Valuable information has been obtained, leading to an increased understanding of the consequences of large releases of radionuclides into the whole environment.

References

Albergel A, Martin D, Strauss B, Gros J-M 1988 The Chernobyl accident: modelling of dispersion over Europe of the radioactive plume and comparison with activity measurements. Atmos Environ 22:2431–2444

Apsimon HM, Wilson J JN 1987 Modeling atmospheric dispersal of the Chernobyl release across Europe. Boundary-Layer Meteorol 41:123–133

Aarkrog A 1969 The direct contamination of rye, barley, wheat and oats with Sr-885, Cs-134, Mn-54 and Ce-141. Radiat Bot 9:357–366

Aarkrog A 1972 Direct contamination of barley with Be-7, Na-22, Cd-115, Sb-125, Cs-134 and Ba-133. Risö-Rep 256:163–175

Bachhuber H, Bunzl K, Dietl F, Schimmak W, Schulz W 1984 Sorption und Ausbreitung von Radionukliden in zwei Ackerböden der Bundesrepublik Deutschland. GSF-Report S-1071, Ingolstädter Landstr. 1, Oberschleissheim

Beresford NA, Mayes RW, Howard BJ et al 1992 The bioavailability of different forms of radiocaesium for transfer across the gut of ruminants. Radiat Prot Dosim 41:87–91

Bonka H, Horn HG, Küppers J, Maqua M 1986 Radiologische Messungen und Strahlenexposition der Bevölkerung Aachen nach dem Reaktorunfall in Tschernobyl. Wiss Umwelt 1:39–50

Borzilov VA, Klepikova NV 1993 Effect of meteorological conditions and release composition on radionuclide deposition after the Chernobyl accident. In: Merwin SE, Balonov MI (eds) The Chernobyl papers, doses to the Soviet population and early health effects studies. Research Enterprises, Richland, WA, p 47–68

Buzulukov YuP, Dobrynin YuL 1993 Release of radionuclides during the Chernobyl accident. In: Merwin SE, Balonov MI (eds) The Chernobyl papers, doses to the Soviet population and early health effects studies. Research Enterprises, Richland, WA, p 3–21

EC 1995 Transfer of radionuclides in animal production systems. Final report of the European Commission Contract F13P-CT920006. European Commission, Brussels

Ertel J, Voigt G, Paretzke HG 1989 Weathering of $^{134/137}$Cs following leaf contamination of grass cultures in an outdoor experiment. Radiat Environ Biophys 28:319–326

Frissel MJ 1992 An update of the recommended soil to plant transfer factors of Sr-90, Cs-137 and transuranics. In: Proc IUR working group meeting 'Soil-to-Plant Transfer Factors', Madrid, Spain, 1–3 June 1992

Garger E, Gordeev S, Holländer W et al 1996 Resuspension and Deposition of radionuclides under various conditions. Proceedings of the 1st International Conference of the European Commission, Belarus, 18–22 March 1996. Russian Federation and Ukraine on the Radiological Consequences of the Chernobyl Accident, Minsk, Belarus

GRS 1987 Neuere Erkenntnisse zum Unfall im Kernkraftwerk Tschernobyl. Gesellschaft für Reaktorsicherheit mbH, Garching (February) p 7–74

Gudiksen PH, Harvey TF, Lange R 1989 Chernobyl source term, atmospheric dispersion, and dose estimation. Health Phys 57:697–706

Hass H, Memmesheimer M, Geiß H, Jakobs HJ, Laube M, Ebel A 1990 Simulation of the Chernobyl radioactive cloud over Europe using the EURAD model. Atmos Environ 24:673A–692A

Hosker RP, Lindberg SE 1982 Atmospheric deposition and plant assimilation of gases and particles. Atmos Environ 16:889–910

ISS 1986 Umweltradioaktivität und Strahlenexposition in Südbayern durch den Tschernonbyl-Unfall. GSF-Institut für Strahlenschutz, Oberschleissheim

Lange R 1978 PATRIC, a three-dimensional particle-in-cell sequential puff code for modeling the transport and diffusion of atmospheric pollutants. Lawrence Livermore National Laboratory, Livermore, CA

Lange R, Dickerson MH, Gudiksen PH 1988 Dose estimates from the Chernobyl accident. Nucl Technol 82:311–322

Middleton LJ 1959 Radioactive strontium and cesium in the edible parts of crops after foliar contamination. Int J Radiat Biol 4:387–402

Müller H, Pröhl G 1988 Cesium transport in food chains: comparison of model predictions and observations. In: Desmet G (ed) Reliability of radioactive transfer models. Elsevier, New York, p 104–112

Müller H, Pröhl G 1993 ECOSYS-87: a dynamic model for assessing radiological consequences of nuclear accidents. Health Phys 64:232–252

Pudykiewicz J 1988 Numerical simulation of the transport of radioactive cloud from the Chernobyl nuclear accident. Tellus 40:241B–259B

Roed J 1987 Dry deposition in rural and in urban areas in Denmark. Radiat Prot Dosim 21:33–36

Selnaes TD, Strand P 1992 Comparison of the uptake of radiocaesium from soil to grass after nuclear weapons tests and the Chernobyl accident. Analyst 117:493–496

Solheim-Hansen H, Hove K 1991 Radiocesium bioavailability: transfer of Chernobyl and tracer radiocesium to goat milk. Health Phys 60:655–673

Tschiersch J, Georgii B 1987 Chernobyl fallout size distribution in urban areas. J Aerosol Sci 18:689–692

Voigt G, Müller H, Pröhl G et al 1989a Experimental determination of transfer coefficients of ^{137}Cs and ^{131}I from fodder into milk of cows and sheep after the Chernobyl accident. Health Phys 57:967–973

Voigt G, Pröhl G, Müller H et al 1989b Determination of the transfer of cesium and iodine from feed into domestic animals. Sci Tot Environ 85:329–338

Voigt G, Pröhl G, Müller H 1991 Experiments on the seasonality of the cesium translocation in cereals, potatoes and vegetables. Radiat Environ Biophys 30:295–303

Voigt G, Howard BJ, Vandecasteele C et al 1993a Factors affecting radiocaesium transfer to ruminants: results of a multinational research group. In: Winter M, Wicke A (eds) Proc 25. Jahrestagung des FfS, Publikationsreihe Fortschritte im Strahlenschutz, Verlag TV Reinland, Köln, p 599–604

Voigt G, Müller H, Paretzke HG, Bauer T, Röhrmoser G 1993b ^{137}Cs transfer after Chernobyl from fodder into chicken meat and eggs. Health Phys 65:141–146

Voigt G, Rauch F, Paretzke HG 1996 Long-term behavior of radiocesium in dairy herds in the years following the Chernobyl accident. Health Phys 71:370–373

Ward GM, Johnson JE 1989 Assessment of milk transfer coefficients for use in prediction models of radioactivity transport. Sci Tot Environ 85:287–294

Wedding JB, Carlson RW, Stukel JJ, Bazzaz FA 1975 Aerosol deposition on plant leaves. Environ Sci Technol 9:151–153

DISCUSSION

Gadd: If your EURAD (EURopean Acid Deposition) model is based on weather forecasting then it is likely to be unreliable, particularly in the short term. You seemed to imply that some of your estimates on precipitation rates were inaccurate because of this.

Voigt: The estimates were not entirely inaccurate. The movement prediction of the rain was too fast so that deposition was predicted to occur at the wrong place. However, if the scale of the world coordinates is shifted, it gives an accurate estimate. This has been checked by measurements. In some respects you are correct, i.e. the model gives a better prediction of long-range effects than short-range ones because the latter is more prone to short-term fluctuations. We are currently trying to improve this by analysing the model assumptions.

Goldman: You have explained the problem relating to wet deposition but there are also large discrepancies in your model for dry deposition. Can you also explain these discrepancies?

Voigt: In the model the deposition velocities were different for day and night, and we found that with this assumption we were obtaining unrealistically high deposition rates during the night. We are now changing the model so that one deposition velocity covers both day and night. The model predictions fit relatively well with the measurements if one deposition velocity is used.

Goldman: The American deposition model, the ARAC (Atmospheric Radiation Advisory Capability) model, located at Lawrence Livermore National Laboratory in California, using a particle-in-cell type of model, predicted the radionuclide concentration of the Chernobyl cloud locations all over the Northern hemisphere within an error factor of two and the arrival date within two days. However, despite these accurate predictions, this model also suffers from the problems of short-range fluctuations. For example, the height of the cloud was underestimated.

Voigt: We also don't know the exact conditions of the source term; for example, the composition of the radionuclides during the release, the height of the source and the temperature of the reactor.

Goldman: The release was not instantaneous: only 25% of the total amount released was released during the first day.

Paretzke: This is not true for the noble gases or for ^{131}I, the bulk of which was most likely released within the first few hours or days. However, ^{137}Cs was released over a longer period (up to eight days), which generates problems if we want to draw conclusions regarding local iodine contaminations (which can no longer be measured) from measured caesium contaminations.

Renn: You showed that there was a three- to fourfold difference between the predicted values and the estimated values for wet deposition. Rather than assuming that your model has made a general over-estimation, is it possible that you just measured at the wrong places?

Voigt: This is a good question because it is a general problem. We are aware that there can be up to a 10-fold difference in single measurements obtained within the same village. Therefore, we have to do some degree of interpolation of measurements within one location and between different locations to account for these differences.

Howard: Many of the deposition measurements are not structured properly. Also, if you take these measurements and interpolate them using geographical techniques you can determine where the greatest uncertainty is and where you should be taking your measurements. This whole field of sampling and measuring procedures in radiation protection is in its infancy compared to many other areas, and we ought to be using up-to-date spatial analysis systems to tell us where we need to sample.

Konoplev: The release at Chernobyl was not homogeneous, and there was a separation of different radionuclide species because of atmospheric dispersion. Therefore, it is not unlikely that fallout at different distances and directions contains radionuclides in different proportions of chemical forms. It follows, therefore, that behaviour, transfer factors and radiological parameters could be different for different places. This situation did not arise for nuclear weapons testing fallout because this was relatively homogeneous. Does your model take this separation into account?

Voigt: No.

Goldman: In practical terms, one of the most interesting observations regarding your data is that most of the dose received by people from contaminated food is a result of initial surface deposition, and that subsequent uptake over the following years is two to three orders of magnitude smaller because of various transport processes. Therefore, a reasonable prediction of the lifetime dose can be made within weeks or months, and concerns about receiving large doses in the future are minimized.

Paretzke: Be careful: we are dealing here only with doses received from ingestion. Fifty per cent of the total dose received by those living in highly contaminated areas comes from external irradiation. In this case the contribution of the first year is of the order of 30% of the time-integrated external dose.

Goldman: But weathering also reduces the dose received by external irradiation.

Håkanson: I have a general philosophical question about the use of transfer coefficients or bio-concentration factors. It is sometimes possible to use transfer coefficients instead of large mechanistic models as a short cut. But transfer coefficients are not constants, they vary between sites and they are time dependent. Therefore, it's a catch-22 situation. Can you comment on this problem, because it also arises in many other contexts?

Voigt: When working with radioecological models, one has to make certain assumptions. There are many factors that influence the transfer of radionuclides to animals and to soil, so the model must be able to adapt to the conditions where it is used. This is especially the case for the animal transfer coefficient, which is commonly used and based on equilibrium conditions. The so-called aggregated transfer factor has also been used. Here, the concentration of radionuclide in the soil is related to the activity concentration in the animal product. Under accidental situations this might be a better estimate than using the fixed transfer coefficient. The ^{137}Cs transfer to milk is now relatively stable and milk activities are close to the levels prior to the Chernobyl accident. However, immediately after the Chernobyl accident, the ^{137}Cs transfer to milk varied by a factor of three or more because of the different deposition scenarios and conditions.

Cigna: All non-linear mechanisms involved in dispersing pollutants are expected to be multifractal processes, which thus justifies the application of multifractal analyses for studying these phenomena. Therefore, a multifractal model may be better at predicting deposition patterns than a more classic model (S. P. Ratti, D. Schertzer, F. Schmitt et al, unpublished results 1994). It is regrettable that the development of this interesting application of fractals to radiation protection is no longer funded in the frame of the 4th Framework Programme of the European Union, Nuclear Fission Safety, 1994–1998, notwithstanding the successful results achieved.

Voigt: We used the EURAD model to predict ^{131}I deposition in Belarus because it is based on weather forecasts. Therefore, it can be applied easily because these data are available, the input values are simple and it predicts the fallout in different countries all over the world. We cross-check these predictions (for ^{137}Cs and ^{131}I) practically in Belarus and Ukraine because it would be useful to have a model that can make quick and reliable short- and long-range predictions after an accident. This model may also be used to predict the dispersion of other pollutants, such as chemicals, which other models are virtually unable to do.

Streffer: What was the ratio between the dose received by plants from deposition and from root uptake?

Voigt: There are many factors that influence the dose received by plants; for example, the charge of the particles or radionuclides. There are differences between the deposition rates of anions and cations, especially during the migration processes of positively and negatively charged ions adhered on leaves through the cuticle, with preference to the uptake of positively charged ions. This process (leaf uptake) is the main contributor to plant contamination shortly after an accident. Root uptake is of minor importance for the following reason. There are differences in the resistance times of radionuclides in the different soil layers, according to the soil characteristics and the chemistry of the radionuclide. For example, the half-life in years per 1 cm layer for the Chernobyl radiocaesium is lower than that from the global fallout radiocaesium. Therefore, Chernobyl radiocaesium could be fixed rapidly and effectively on clay minerals and humic acids. According to more recent investigations (K. Bunzl, personal communication 1996) in a German soil more than 70% is no longer available for root uptake and subsequent transfer into plants. In the case of ^{131}I, due to its short half-life (eight days) only uptake by leaves and plant-adhered ^{131}I is of importance when considering the dose to humans.

Streffer: What was the chemical form of the iodine when it was deposited several kilometres away from the source?

Voigt: About 40–50% of iodine was deposited in the form of aerosols, which were 0.1–1.0 mm in diameter. About 25–30% was in a gaseous form as elemental iodine and 25–30% was in an organically bound form.

Goldman: Are insoluble particles that are not taken up by plants and animals incorporated in your model?

Voigt: No.

Frissel: I have a comment and a question. It is possible to model the migration of radionuclides such as caesium, strontium, plutonium and americum in soil relatively well. The migration rates in agricultural soils vary between 0.1 cm/y for plutonium to 0.5 cm/y for strontium, and for caesium 0.3 cm/y is a good estimate. The uncertainty is relatively low, but there are exceptions depending on soil type or rain intensity.

My question is that if it is estimated that the predicted uptake of radionuclides from soils by plants is within a factor of 10 of the measured value, what should we expect from an assessment model in general? How accurate would it be at predicting the consequences of a large release of radionuclides at unknown locations; for example, in South America?

Voigt: These models have been created to make estimates under mainly European conditions or at least in the Northern hemisphere. We have attempted to apply our ECOSYS radioecology model to other climatic conditions, such as in Hong Kong and Korea, and it works well after adaptation. The most important point is that all these models can make reliable estimates for the conditions for which they were designed, but it remains to be proven how accurate they would be at predicting an accident in South America, for example, after adapting them to the local circumstances. Using these models without modifications, however, would result in wrong predictions.

Whicker: You mentioned that the increase in the transfer coefficient of radiocaesium to animal products with time was due to a general breakdown of the more insoluble particles. How do you interpret this?

Voigt: The low milk transfer coefficient of ^{137}Cs in 1986 and 1987 was presumably due to a direct contamination on leaves after radionuclides. This ^{137}Cs has a different chemical form compared to the ^{137}Cs incorporated into plant material after root uptake. At the GSF Institut für Strahlenschutz we have observed a change in milk transfer during the years. Other groups have also reported an increased transfer coefficient with time. It is possible that temporal and spatial changes in resuspension are involved.

Whicker: Does the extractability of radiocaesium from the soil change with time?

Paretzke: Yes, this might well be the case. But these measurements reported here were made in the grass of the same area, so they would be influenced by changes in extractability only slowly, i.e. in years, and not during shorter periods (e.g. during one or two months).

Voigt: In 1993 we monitored the ^{137}Cs activities in milk and vegetation samples from a Bavarian farm by taking measurements every second day. We found that the activities of the vegetation samples varied considerably, but that the levels of radiocaesium in milk were rather invariable.

Gadd: You mentioned the transport of radiocaesium in the soil, but you did not mention the role of micro-organisms, which have important roles in all soils, in these transport processes. Are the roles of micro-organisms included in your model?

Voigt: That's a good question. Presently we have restricted our studies to agricultural areas for the reason that there are less confounding factors, such as microflora, which play a more important role in areas such as forests or semi-natural environments.

The radioecological significance of semi-natural ecosystems

B. J. Howard and D. C. Howard

Institute of Terrestrial Ecology, Merlewood Research Station, Grange-over-Sands, Cumbria LA11 6JU, UK

Abstract. The transfer of radiocaesium to many food products either produced in or harvested from semi-natural ecosystems is high compared with intensive agricultural areas. Radiocaesium contamination levels in semi-natural foods are highly variable and difficult to predict. Spatial analysis may help to explain some of the variability and give improved estimates of the total output of radiocaesium in food products produced or harvested from semi-natural ecosystems. Consumption of foodstuffs from semi-natural ecosystems can contribute significantly to radiocaesium ingestion by humans. The long effective half-lives that occur for some semi-natural products lead to an increase with time in their importance compared with agricultural products. In determining the importance of semi-natural food products, the diet needs to be considered for both the average population and for special groups who utilize these environments to a greater extent than normal. Effective countermeasures have been developed to reduce radiocaesium levels in some semi-natural products.

1997 Health impacts of large releases of radionuclides. Wiley, Chichester (Ciba Foundation Symposium 203) p 21–43

The aim of this chapter is to consider the transfer of radiocaesium to food from semi-natural ecosystems, to assess the importance of such ecosystems as a source of radiocaesium intake by humans and to summarize the available countermeasures for these ecosystems. A novel approach to quantifying the radionuclide movement in and from semi-natural ecosystems is discussed.

Semi-natural ecosystems as discussed here include non-intensively managed areas such as forests, heathlands, uplands and mountain pastures, marshlands and tundra. A variety of different foodstuffs — including fungi, berries, honey, meat from a range of different domesticated and game animals, and milk — are taken from these ecosystems.

Contamination of semi-natural ecosystems

The potential importance of semi-natural ecosystems compared with agricultural areas in producing food products with high radiocaesium activity concentrations became evident in the period of above ground nuclear weapons testing. Radiocaesium contamination of reindeer/caribou (*Rangifer rangifer*) in many countries was much higher than that of agricultural animals, with reported activity concentrations exceeding $1000 \, \text{Bq kg}^{-1}$ fresh weight. Activity concentrations in the order of tens to thousands of Bq kg^{-1} fresh weight were also recorded for various other deer species, moose (*Alces alces*) (Howard et al 1991) and mushrooms (on a dry weight basis) (Grüter 1971).

Fallout from the Chernobyl accident was deposited on many semi-natural ecosystems in Europe due to their higher rates of precipitation. Intervention limits for radiocaesium have been exceeded for many semi-natural products in different European countries.

Transfer to semi-natural food products

A common method used to quantify transfer of radiocaesium to semi-natural products is to calculate the aggregated transfer coefficient (T_{ag}), defined as the activity concentration in the product (in Bq kg^{-1} fresh or dry weight) divided by the deposition rate (in Bq m^{-2}) (Howard et al 1996). T_{ag} values are not appropriate for the period immediately following deposition, and they are most useful when combined with information on the rate of reduction in contamination levels in various products. This is commonly quantified using the effective half-life, T_{ef}, which describes the time required for the activity concentration of a radionuclide in a food product to be reduced to one half of the original concentration in a specific system, and therefore the T_{ef} incorporates physical decay. T_{ag} values have recently been collated (Howard et al 1996) and therefore a comparison of transfer values will not be attempted here. In general, aggregated transfer rates decline in the following order:

$$\text{mushrooms} \gg \text{reindeer} > \text{berries} > \text{game} > \text{domesticated animals.}$$

However, the considerable variability in transfer rates leads to exceptions to this general trend. There are large differences between the fruiting bodies of different fungal species (for simplicity termed mushrooms), where threefold differences in T_{ag} values occur. A number of species-specific and environmental characteristics contribute to the high and variable radiocaesium levels in semi-natural products. These have been summarized by Howard et al (1996) and in a recent Nordic radioecology publication (Dahlgaard 1994). These are used as a basis for the following brief outline.

Interception and retention on plant surfaces

The rate of interception by plant surfaces is highly variable in semi-natural ecosystems, depending on factors such as biomass and the presence of coniferous or deciduous tree stands. Interception of radiocaesium can therefore range from below 5% of the total deposited on heavily grazed pastures in mountain areas with low vegetation biomass to more than 50% in semi-natural pasture (Livens et al 1992) and 60–100% in dense coniferous forest (e.g. Tikhomirov & Shcheglov 1991). The effect of high interception rates on radiocaesium levels in semi-natural food products is limited, especially over the longer term, except for lichen. In thick lichen mats interception is nearly complete and the original deposit can be retained over many years. The ability of lichens to intercept and retain radiocaesium is radioecologically significant because of its role as a major food source for reindeer/caribou.

Soil properties

The uptake of radiocaesium from soils in semi-natural ecosystems was not extensively studied before the Chernobyl accident possibly because the fallout from atmospheric weapons testing was deposited continuously onto plant surfaces over a long period, thereby masking the importance of root uptake. Nevertheless, the high uptake of ^{137}Cs from upper soil layers with a high organic matter content was noted (Barber 1964). The low capacity of many of the soil types characteristic of semi-natural ecosystems to immobilize radiocaesium is one of the main factors responsible for the continued high radiocaesium levels in plants and animals. A soil allowing a high rate of root uptake of radiocaesium has been characterized in northern Europe as typically having a low clay and potassium content, a low pH, and a high organic matter content (Livens & Loveland 1988). Radiocaesium is not strongly bound to the soil components; consequently it is available for uptake from the soil solution (see Desmet et al 1991 for review). Nevertheless, radiocaesium usually migrates slowly down the soil profile and remains for long periods in the upper soil layers where root biomass is greatest.

Radiocaesium uptake by vegetation is also affected by the rate at which it moves down the soil profile. For example, Beresford et al (1992) found that T_{ag} values for Chernobyl ^{137}Cs in vegetation in upland ecosystems in the UK were higher than those for pre-Chernobyl [137]Cs ('aged deposits'). They attributed this to the greater depth of the 'aged deposit', over 50% of which was below the 0–4 cm layer down the soil profile and therefore out of the rooting zone of the vegetation. Distribution of radiocaesium in the soil profile will obviously affect T_{ag} values that are based on total deposition.

Fungal uptake of radiocaesium

Fungal hyphae are usually confined to the upper organic horizons of the soil. Assessments of fungal biomass and measurements of radiocaesium uptake by hyphae suggest that a high proportion of deposited radiocaesium may be present in the fungal mycelium (Olsen et al 1990, Dighton et al 1991), and this may account to some extent for the observed retention of radiocaesium in the upper layers of organic soils.

The highest radiocaesium activity concentrations reported in food products since the Chernobyl accident have been in mushrooms. Radiocaesium activity concentrations in some species (e.g. *Cantharellus cibarius* and *Leccinum testaceoscabrum*) are comparable with higher plants growing in the same area. In contrast, in other species radiocaesium activity concentrations are 10–100-fold higher than those of higher plants (e.g. *Rozites caperatus*, *Suillus variegatus* and *Lactarius rufus*) (Bakken & Olsen 1990, Haselwandter et al 1988).

Radiocaesium uptake by vegetation

The proportion of radiocaesium that resides in the vegetation of semi-natural ecosystems is often much greater than that which occurs in agricultural ecosystems. This is due to two factors: (i) increased plant uptake due to soil properties; and (ii) the ability of certain herbaceous species, notably ericoid dwarf shrubs, to accumulate higher levels of radiocaesium than other plants. Berries of ericoid dwarf shrubs that can accumulate high levels of radiocaesium include bilberries (*Vaccinium myrtillus*) and lingonberries (*Vaccinium vitis-idaea*) (Johanson et al 1991). In addition, heather (*Calluna vulgaris*) has been shown to have an order of magnitude higher radiocaesium activity concentration than adjacent herbaceous plants (Bunzl & Kracke 1986, Horrill et al 1995). In Germany heather honey was found to be nearly 100-fold more contaminated than flower honey (Bunzl et al 1988), and radiocaesium levels in sheep on heather moorland were elevated compared with other ecosystems (Bunzl & Kracke 1984).

Radiocaesium levels in vascular plants can be ranked in the following order: ericoid dwarf shrubs > herbs > grasses > shrubs and trees (Horrill et al 1990); however, there are many exceptions.

Dietary preferences and grazing behaviour of animals

Herbivores vary widely in their feeding habits in semi-natural ecosystems. In addition to differences in feed selection between animal species, seasonal differences in the available forage plants contribute markedly to variation in radiocaesium activity concentrations in animals. The high radiocaesium activity concentrations reported for animals in many semi-natural ecosystems are due to the high radiocaesium levels in the vegetation species eaten by animals combined with the comparatively high transfer of radiocaesium to small ruminant species — such as sheep (*Ovis aries*), goats (*Capra hircus*) and roe-deer (*Capreolus capreolus*) — that frequently occur in these ecosystems (see Howard et al 1991 for review).

Variation in dietary preferences between seasons leads to substantial differences in radiocaesium levels in some animals, notably reindeer and roe-deer. However, radiocaesium intake is determined by both the contamination concentrations and total daily herbage intake, and it has been shown that when moose change to a more contaminated diet there is also a concomitant reduction in overall herbage intake which would reduce the effect of a diet change on total radiocaesium consumption (Johanson 1994). The consumption of mushrooms in autumn has been found to lead to autumnal peaks in radiocaesium levels in many animal species, including sheep (Hove et al 1990) and roe-deer (Johanson 1994). For instance, in Norway the transfer of radiocaesium to goat milk increased two- to fourfold in those years with a comparatively high fungal abundance (Hove et al 1990).

In winter lichens form the major part (70–80%) of the diet of reindeer and therefore radiocaesium levels in reindeer rise considerably during this season. The ^{137}Cs activity concentrations in reindeer during summer and early autumn are generally only about 10–20% of the winter values because radiocaesium activity concentrations in other vegetation are generally considerably lower than those of lichens. This situation has persisted for at least nine years following the Chernobyl accident. Therefore, a lichen intake during the summer of only 10–20% dry weight will determine radiocaesium levels in reindeer meat (Gaare & Staaland 1994).

Diet selection is also important in determining radiocaesium levels in birds. For instance, radiocaesium levels in red grouse (*Lapogus lapogus scoticus*) and black grouse (*Tetrao tetrix*) in Scotland were higher after the Chernobyl accident than those in willow grouse (*Lapogus lapogus*) in Nordic countries. This is because the grouse in Scotland eat large quantities of heather, which does not form an important part of the diet of willow grouse.

Radiocaesium levels in both moose and roe-deer have been found to be lower when these animals have access to farmland where herbage with lower contamination levels is available (Johanson 1994).

Long-term changes in contamination levels

Although radiocaesium activity concentrations in agricultural products declined relatively rapidly after the Chernobyl accident, those in many natural food products did not. The prime reason for the high radiocaesium levels in semi-natural fungi, plants and animals, with the notable exception of reindeer, is the persistently high rates of uptake of radiocaesium from soil. As with transfer of radiocaesium there are substantial differences reported in effective half-lives with food types and within species from different types of semi-natural ecosystem. For some species in semi-natural ecosystems quantifiable declines have been recorded in radiocaesium activity concentrations since the Chernobyl accident. However, there are notable exceptions, including moose, roe-deer (Johanson 1994) and various species of mushrooms. If there is no measurable decrease with time the physical half-life of ^{137}Cs will determine the effective half-life. The long effective half-lives compared with many agricultural food products lead to an increase in the comparative importance of food products from semi-natural ecosystems with time.

The effects of human dietary preferences on radiocaesium ingestion rates

The importance of semi-natural ecosystems as a source of human radiocaesium contamination received little attention prior to the Chernobyl accident, with the notable exception of the reindeer/caribou herders. The implicit assumption was that the quantities of food consumed from these systems were small and confined to a small proportion of the population in most countries. They were therefore usually not considered in dose assessments.

The potential importance of semi-natural ecosystems became apparent after the Chernobyl accident because in some of the most heavily contaminated areas semi-natural food products form an important component of the diet. A number of different studies have been carried out with the aim of quantifying the importance of food produced or harvested in semi-natural ecosystems as sources of radiocaesium to different population groups (Strand et al 1989, Aarkrog 1994).

In some countries there are certain common foodstuffs that are of particular concern. A good example are whey cheeses produced from goat milk (Norwegian brown cheese). Such cheeses can have comparatively high radiocaesium levels because manufacturing involves evaporation of the whey to dryness, which increases the radiocaesium activity concentration by a factor of about 10.

Recently, a detailed study has been conducted to compare the importance of different food sources in determining the radiocaesium ingestion by village residents in areas contaminated by the Chernobyl accident in Ukraine and Russia (ECP9, Strand et al 1996). The study combined measurements of contamination levels in foodstuffs with dietary surveys and whole-body measurements. Consumption of forest products was usually small, in weight and energy terms, compared to the consumption of foods derived from private or collective farming. However, the transfer of radiocaesium to semi-natural products, such as mushrooms, berries, fish and game, was considerably higher than in agricultural systems. For all the study sites assessed, one-third to a half of the population consumed mushrooms and berries. However, the consumption of game was infrequent. For all study sites, a strong relationship was found between the extent of mushroom consumption reported and whole-body radiocaesium content (Fig. 1).

Food sources were divided into three categories in order to identify sources and pathways leading to intake of radiocaesium by the rural population. These were: (i) collective farming/state shop; (ii) private farming; and (iii) semi-natural products. An initial estimate has been made of the average contribution of each food production system to internal dose of the rural population by combining results from the dietary survey with the measurements of radiocaesium levels in food (Fig. 2). At the Russian site there was a compulsory sale of private cattle in 1986, and therefore private milk was not available to most people.

At the Russian site natural food products were the main contributors to radiocaesium intake, whilst at the Ukrainian site food from private farming was the most important. At both study sites it was apparent that consumption of natural produce was an important contributor to internal dose, and mushrooms were the main natural food influencing intake of radiocaesium. In both republics an average of more than 90% of radiocaesium intake attributed to natural food products was due to mushrooms.

On a larger scale Nielsen (1995) has attempted to make an initial comparison of the importance of agricultural and semi-natural products for a number of different European countries. The average individual doses arising from the consumption of Chernobyl ^{137}Cs in food products from agricultural and semi-natural food products was estimated by combining information on average consumption rates of major foodstuffs with relevant transfer coefficients and effective half-lives. Foodstuffs considered included

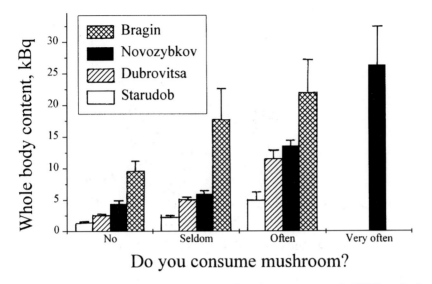

FIG. 1.   Radiocaesium body burdens in groups of mushroom eaters at the ECP9 study sites (Skuterud et al 1996). Bragin, Novozybkov and Starudob are in Russia. Dubrovitsa is in the Ukraine.

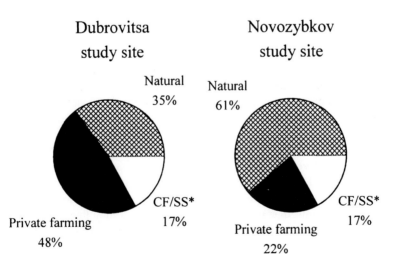

FIG. 2.   Comparative importance of different food production systems for the intake of radiocaesium at the ECP9 study sites in Ukraine (Dubrovitsa) and Russia (Novozybkov). CF/SS*, collective farm/state shop (Strand et al 1996).

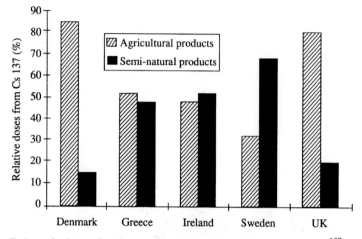

FIG. 3.   Estimated relative distribution of calculated doses from ingestion of ^{137}Cs from the Chernobyl accident produced in agricultural and semi-natural areas in different European countries (Nielsen 1995).

milk and grain products, potatoes, vegetables, fruit, beef, pork, game, freshwater fish, mushrooms and lamb/mutton. The relative distributions of the doses from ingestion of ^{137}Cs from agricultural and semi-natural ecosystems are shown in Fig. 3. The comparative importance of the two sources varies considerably between countries with Denmark and the UK receiving the highest dose from agricultural products, whereas the reverse occurs in Sweden. The authors acknowledged the preliminary nature of the data, and emphasized the need to consider a wider range of foodstuffs and to improve the estimates, particularly regarding information on variation in the average and maximal amounts consumed of different components of the diet.

The consumption of foodstuffs from semi-natural ecosystems can significantly contribute to radiocaesium ingestion by humans. In determining the importance of this route it is necessary to consider the diet of both the average population and that of special groups who utilize these environments to a greater extent than normal.

Predicting radiocaesium levels in food from semi-natural ecosystems

Models have been developed for agricultural systems that predict the transfer of radionuclides to food products with an acceptable degree of accuracy. However, modelling such transfers to food and finally to humans is much more difficult for semi-natural ecosystems due to the many factors that can influence the fate of radionuclides in these complex ecosystems: deposition tends to be more heterogeneous, and there is also a pronounced heterogeneity in soil properties and a much higher variability in dietary selection and grazing ranges of food-producing animals compared with agriculturally improved areas. Therefore, a consistent characteristic of semi-natural foods is a high interspecies and intraspecies variability in radiocaesium activity concentrations.

Although general statements can be made about the high rates of transfer and long effective half-lives for semi-natural foods, there will be many exceptions to such statements. Estimates of the total export of radiocaesium from semi-natural ecosystems, based on large-scale production values or dietary intake estimates and generic transfer values, are likely to have a high degree of uncertainty associated with them. If the regional variation in transfer, production/harvesting and dietary preferences can be incorporated then it might be possible to provide improved estimates of the net output and ingestion of radiocaesium in semi-natural products.

The value of spatial analysis of important parameters can be demonstrated by considering the transfer of radiocaesium to red grouse, which is managed as a game bird in heather moorland in upland areas of Great Britain. After the Chernobyl accident, radiocaesium activity concentrations in red grouse in Scotland were higher than any other product. There are three reasons for this: (i) the high rates of transfer of radiocaesium to heather compared with other herbaceous species; (ii) the preferred diet of the birds, which is almost exclusively young heather shoots: and (iii) the high rate of transfer which occurs from heather to grouse meat. Recent studies on this ecosystem have provided transfer data for radiocaesium uptake by heather on the two major soil types in heather moorland, peat and peaty podsol soils (Horrill et al 1995), and an estimate of the transfer coefficient for grouse meat (Moss & Horrill 1996). These data have been combined with spatial information on grouse and dense heath distribution to give information on the likely geographical variation in transfer of radiocaesium to grouse meat (B. J. Howard, D. C. Howard, V. H. Kennedy & R. W. Moss, unpublished observations 1996).

Aggregated transfer coefficients for the current years growth of heather were made in 1990. The values used for the spatial analysis were 0.27 and 0.76 $m^2 kg^{-1}$ dry weight for peaty podsol and peat soils, respectively. The transfer of radiocaesium to meat is often quantified using the transfer coefficient, defined as the equilibrium ratio between the activity concentration in the meat ($Bq kg^{-1}$ fresh weight) divided by the daily intake of activity ($Bq d^{-1}$) (Ward & Johnson 1986). In controlled conditions Moss & Horrill (1996) measured a transfer coefficient for radiocaesium transfer to grouse meat of $10 d kg^{-1}$. By combining the above estimates of radiocaesium transfer from soil to current heather growth and hence to grouse meat the radiocaesium activity concentration in grouse meat for the two different soil types was predicted for different deposition rates of radiocaesium (Fig. 4). The estimate assumes that the grouse are feeding exclusively on current heather growth and are consuming $55 g d^{-1}$.

As the two soil types are spatially distinct some form of geographical framework can be built into a predictive model. The distribution of peat and podsol, as recorded by the Soil Survey and Land Research Centre (SSLRC) and Macaulay Land Use Research Institute (MLURI) is shown in Fig. 5a. Grouse are not evenly distributed across Great Britain, and their presence and population density are recorded by the British Trust for Ornithology (BTO). A distribution map is shown in Fig. 5b; the information is recorded for tetrads (2 km × 2 km), which can be refined using the known

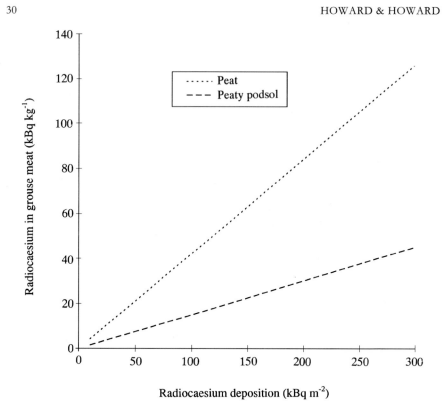

FIG. 4.   Predicted radiocaesium content of grouse meat on contrasting soil types for different rates of deposited radiocaesium.

distribution of dense heath. The Institute of Terrestrial Ecology Land Cover Map of Great Britain (Barr et al 1993) is a satellite-derived map that identifies dense shrub heath as a category, and its distribution is shown in Fig. 5c. Spatial overlay allows the coincidence of these three elements to be identified (Fig. 6a).

In Great Britain grouse are only usually shot on estates that are managed for their production. The numbers of grouse shot are recorded for each estate and published for regions (Fig. 6b, Hudson 1992). The proportion of each region's harvest, which have fed on heather on different soil types, can be estimated by using the ratio of grouse present on dense heath growing over peat and podsol as a weighting factor. There are a number of assumptions made when using this ratio, both about the quality and appropriateness of the different data sets. Assuming the average meat content of harvested grouse is 200 g per carcass and that deposition was a uniform 100 kBq/m^2, the total body burden of radiocaesium for one harvest season can be calculated. Its distribution is shown in Fig. 6c.

The analysis thus gives a predicted spatial distribution in total ^{137}Cs output in red grouse meat for each region. Considerable variation occurs in population numbers of

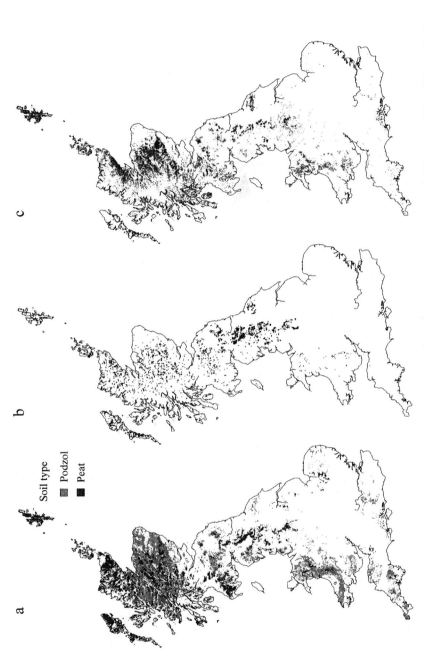

FIG. 5. (a) The soil types shown are peat and podsol, mapped at 1 km² resolution. Data sources are the Soil Survey and Land Research Centre (SSLRC) for England and Wales and the Macaulay Land Use Research Institute (MLURI) for Scotland. (b) the presence of grouse between 1988 and 1991 (recorded per tetrad). The data source is the British Trust for Ornithology (BTO). (c) Dart areas indicate the presence of dense health. Data taken from the Institute of Terrestrial Ecology Land Cover Map of Great Britain.

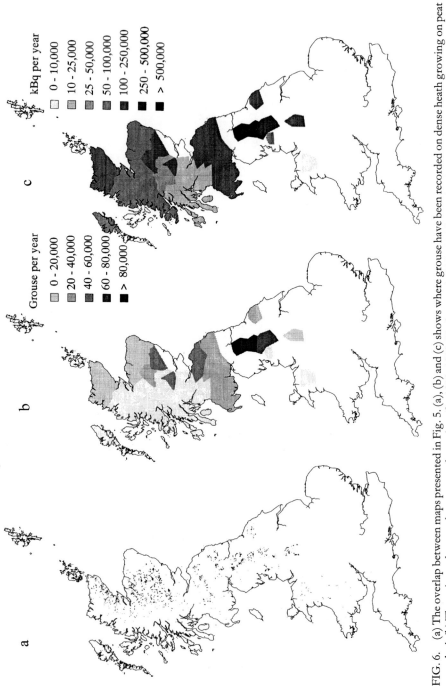

FIG. 6. (a) The overlap between maps presented in Fig. 5. (a), (b) and (c) shows where grouse have been recorded on dense heath growing on peat or podsol. (b) The estimated grouse bag per year by regions for 1970–1989 (Hudson et al 1992). (c) The total radiocaesium output in grouse by region calculated assuming a deposition of 100 kBq/m².

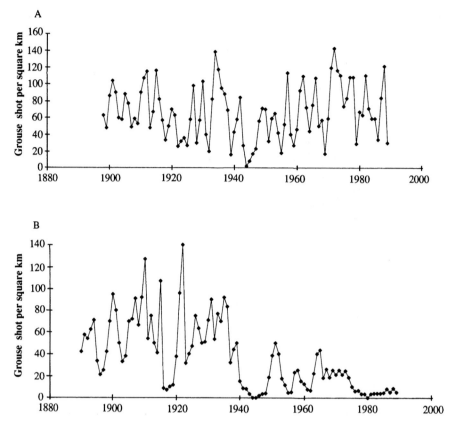

FIG. 7.   Examples of the temporal variation in grouse harvests in different areas of Great Britain (from Hudson 1992): (A) Cumbria and North Dales; and (B) Moray and Nairn.

red grouse, and therefore total production of red grouse (Fig. 7) and flux of radiocaesium, will also vary accordingly.

The example for red grouse, although limited to only two soil types, demonstrates several general aspects of such spatial analysis:

(1)   information is needed on the spatial distribution of the semi-natural products;
(2)   transfer values are needed which reflect the spatial variation of the major controlling variables;
(3)   if regional production (or harvesting) rates of the semi-natural products are taken into account then improved estimates of net flux of radiocaesium can be calculated;

(4)   temporal variation in many semi-natural populations occurs, and this will affect total flux of radiocaesium, and hence total radiocaesium intake by consumers; and

(5)   combining information on transfer and fluxes of radiocaesium with information on movement of foodstuffs and dietary habits has the potential to give improved estimates of radiocaesium transfer to special groups.

Spatial analysis allows a spatial structure to be applied to process models. One benefit from the approach is that it focuses attention not only on radiocaesium transfer values, but also on production and consumption data requirements, which also have an important influence on total radiocaesium movement both within and exported from semi-natural ecosystems. Further consideration needs to be given to the approach, including the ways in which uncertainties in the predictions can be derived and presented, and on how changes with time are incorporated.

Countermeasures

The application of countermeasures to reduce radiocaesium contamination of food products from semi-natural ecosystems has been the subject of considerable attention in the 10 years since the Chernobyl accident. Whilst highly effective countermeasures have been developed for agricultural products, their use in semi-natural ecosystems is hampered by difficulties in applying the countermeasure appropriately. Although it is relatively easy to apply ameliorants such as potassium fertilizers to arable fields or pastures, their application in mountainous or forested areas is more difficult. Furthermore, the ecological side-effects in some semi-natural environments may be adversely affected by widespread application of such ameliorants.

Suitable countermeasures for semi-natural ecosystems have been reviewed by Hove (1993) and Howard (1993). The simplest countermeasure for contaminated animals is the provision of uncontaminated feed or pasture. For most domesticated ruminants 'clean feeding' effectively reduces radiocaesium burdens with a half-life varying between 10–40 days, depending on the species. Clean feeding is labour intensive and expensive and therefore caesium binders, such as clay minerals and hexacyanoferrate compounds, have also been widely used since the Chernobyl accident. Caesium binders must be present in the gastrointestinal tract continuously, and at adequately high concentrations, in order to be effective. Many of the animals in semi-natural ecosystems are handled infrequently, if at all, and therefore it is not possible to give them daily doses of caesium binders. For semi-domesticated, free-ranging animals two main methods have been developed to deliver the binder to the animal: rumen-dwelling boli and salt licks. The rumen-dwelling boli, developed in Norway, are composed of compressed ammonium hexacyanoferrate (AFCF), barite and wax and gradually release the AFCF binder into the gastrointestinal tract. Hove & Hansen (1993) reported that the presence of one, two or three boli reduced radiocaesium activity concentrations in sheep milk by 35%, 60% and 85%, respectively. The reduction effect persisted for 90 days, but with a reduced efficiency. Recently, additions of a wax coating to the boli have been made to delay the onset of binder release and maximize the reduction effect in the period prior to the recovery of treated animals (Hansen et al 1996). A salt lick with 2.5% AFCF has also been developed for use in mountain pastures in Norway. The salt licks are placed in contaminated areas where animals are accustomed to using them as a source of additional sodium. In Norway the use of salt licks is estimated to achieve an average reduction in radiocaesium levels in meat of about 50% (Hove 1993). However, the efficiency of licks depends on the frequency at which animals use them, and some animals will not use the licks at all. It is therefore important to combine the use of AFCF salt licks, and indeed other countermeasures, with live monitoring.

Whilst the countermeasures listed above are suitable for domestic or semi-domestic animals, they are of little use for game, although the possible use of salt licks has been considered. Few measures are possible for these animals, although changes in the hunting season, and ensuring that mobile, live-monitoring stations are available for measurement of carcasses, can lead to reductions in radiocaesium intake via game (Howard 1993).

For forest products such as mushrooms and berries there are no practical countermeasures available that can be applied *in situ*. However, advice about food preparation procedures such as soaking or boiling mushrooms can lead to considerable reductions of around 90% in their radiocaesium content. In addition, public information campaigns to inform people about which species are the most contaminated could substantially reduce radiocaesium intake rates via mushrooms.

Acknowledgements

This review was conducted as an initial exercise under the European Commission fourth framework programme, Spatial Analysis of Vulnerable Ecosystems (SAVE), Contract F14P-CT95–0015. We thank many colleagues at the Institute of Terrestrial Ecology, including C. Naylor, V. Kennedy, R. Moss, C. Barnett and N. Beresford.

References

Aarkrog A 1994 Doses from the Chernobyl accident to the Nordic populations via diet intake. In: Dahlgaard H (ed) Nordic radioecology. The transfer of radionuclides through Nordic ecosystems to man. Elsevier, Amsterdam, p 433–456 (Studies in Environ Sci Ser 62)

Bakken LR, Olsen R 1990 Accumulation of radiocaesium in fungi. Can J Microbiol 36:704–710

Barber DA 1964 Influence of soil organic matter on the entry of caesium-137 into plants. Nature 204:1326–1327

Barr CJ, Bunce RGH, Clarke RT et al 1993 Countryside survey 1990: main report. Countryside 1990, vol 2. Department of the Environment, London

Beresford NA, Howard BJ, Barnett CL, Crout NMJ 1992 The uptake by vegetation of Chernobyl and aged radiocaesium in upland west Cumbria. J Environ Radiat 16:181–195

Bunzl K, Kracke W 1984 Fallout $^{239/240}$ Pu and ^{137} Cs in animal livers consumed by man. Health Phys 46:466–470

Bunzl K, Kracke W 1986 Accumulation of fallout ^{137}Cs in some plants and berries of the family Ericaceae. Health Phys 50:540–542

Bunzl K, Kracke W, Vorwhol G 1988 Transfer of Chernobyl-derived [134]Cs, ^{137}Cs, ^{131}I and [103]Ru from flowers to honey and pollen. J Environ Radiat 6:261–269

Dahlgaard H 1994 Nordic radioecology. The transfer of radionuclides through Nordic ecosystems to man. Elsevier, Amsterdam (Studies in Environ Sci Ser 62)

Desmet GM, Van Loon LR, Howard BJ 1991 Chemical speciation and bioavailability of elements in the environment and their relevance to radioecology. Sci Total Environ 100:105–124

Dighton J, Clint GM, Poskitt J 1991 Uptake and accumulation of ^{137}Cs by upland grassland soil fungi: a potential pool of Cs immobilization. Mycol Res 95:1052–1056

Gaare E, Staaland H 1994 Pathways of fallout radiocaesium via reindeer to man. In: Dahlgaard H (ed) Nordic radioecology. The transfer of radionuclides through Nordic ecosystems to man. Elsevier, Amsterdam, p 303–334 (Studies in Environ Sci Ser 62)

Grüter H 1971 Radioactive fission product ^{137}Cs in mushrooms in west Germany during 1963–1970. Health Phys 20:655–656

Hansen HS, Hove K, Barvik K 1996 The effect of sustained release boli with ammoniumiron (III)–hexacyanoferrate(II) on radiocesium accumulation in sheep grazing contaminated pasture. Health Phys 71:705–712

Haselwandter K, Berreck M, Brunner P 1988 Fungi as bioindicators of radiocaesium contamination: pre- and post- Chernobyl activities. Trans Br Mycol Soc 90:171–174

Horrill AD, Kennedy VH, Harwood TR 1990 The concentrations of Chernobyl-derived radionuclides in species characteristic of natural and semi-natural ecosystems. In: Desmet G (ed) Transfer of radionuclides in natural and semi-natural environments. Elsevier, Oxon, p 27–39

Horrill AD, Patterson IS, Miller GR et al 1995 Studies on radiocaesium transfer in heather dominant ecosystems. Final report Scottish Development Department. Institute of Terrestrial Ecology, Grange-over-Sands

Hove K 1993 Chemical methods for reduction of the transfer of radionuclides to farm animals in semi-natural ecosystems. Sci Total Environ 137:235–248

Hove K, Hansen HS 1993 Reduction of radiocaesium transfer of animal products using sustained release boli with ammoniumiron(III)hexacyanoferrate(II). Acta Vet Scand 34:287–297

Hove K, Pedersen O, Garmo TH, Hansen HS, Staaland H 1990 Fungi: a major source of radiocaesium contamination of grazing ruminants in Norway. Health Phys 59:189–192

Howard BJ 1993 Management methods of reducing radionuclide contamination of animal food products in semi-natural ecosystems. Sci Total Environ 137:249–260

Howard BJ, Beresford NA, Hove K 1991 Transfer of radiocesium to ruminants in unimproved natural and semi-natural ecosystems and appropriate countermeasures. Health Phys 61:715–725

Howard BJ, Johanson K, Linsley GS, Hove K, Pröhl G, Horyna J 1996 Transfer of radionuclides by terrestrial food products from semi-natural ecosystems to man. Second report of the VAMP Terrestrial Working Group, IAEA-TECDOC-857 p 47–49, International Atomic Energy Agency, Vienna

Hudson P 1992 Grouse in space and time. The population biology of a managed gamebird. Game Conservancy Ltd, Hampshire

Johanson KJ 1994 Radiocaesium in game animals in the Nordic countries. In: Dahlgaard H (ed) Nordic radioecology. Studies in environmental science 62: The transfer of radionuclides through Nordic ecosystems to man. Elsevier, Amsterdam, p 287–301

Johanson KJ, Bergstrom R, Von Bothmer S, Kardell L 1991 Radiocaesium in Swedish forest ecosystems. In: Moberg L (ed) The Chernobyl fallout in Sweden. Swedish Radiation Protection Institute, Stockholm, p 477–486

Livens FR, Loveland PJ 1988 The influence of soil properties on the environmental mobility. Soil Use Manage 4:69–75

Livens FR, Fowler D, Horrill AD 1992 Wet and dry deposition of I-131, Cs-134 and Cs-137 at an upland site in northern Britain. J Environ Radiat 16:243–254

Moss RW, Horrill AD 1996 Metabolism of radiocaesium in red grouse. J Environ Radiat 33:49–62

Nielsen S 1995 Dose from Cs-137 in food produced in semi natural environments. In: McGarry A (ed) Radioecology of semi-natural ecosystems. Final report Sep 1992–June 1995, Commission of the European Communities. Radiation Protection Institute of Ireland, Dublin

Olsen RA, Joner E, Bakken LR 1990 Soil fungi and the fate of radiocaesium in the soil ecosystem: a discussion of possible mechanisms involved in the radiocaesium accumulation in fungi and the role of fungi as a Cs sink in the soil. In: Desmet G (ed) Transfer of radionuclides in natural and semi-natural environments. Elsevier, Oxon, p 657–663

Skuterud L, Travnikova I, Balanov M, Strand P, Howard BJ 1996 Importance of fungi for intake of radiocaesium by populations in Russia. Sci Total Environ, in press

Strand P, Bøe E, Berteig L et al 1989 Whole-body counting and dietary surveys in Norway during the first year after the Chernobyl accident. Radiat Prot Dosim 27:163–171

Strand P, Howard BJ, Averin V 1996 Transfer of radionuclides to animals, their comparative importance under different agricultural ecosystems and appropriate countermeasures. Experimental collaboration project no. 9: final report. International scientific collaboration on the consequences of the Chernobyl accident (1991–1995). European Commission, Belarus, the Russian Federation, Ukraine. EUR 16539EN. European Commission, Luxembourg

Tikhomirov FA, Shcheglov AI 1991 The Radiological consequences of the Kyshtym and Chernobyl radiation accidents for forest ecosystems. Seminar on comparative assessment of the environmental impact of radionuclides released during three major nuclear accidents: Kyshtym, Windscale, Chernobyl. EUR 13574 867–887 Commission of the European Communities, Luxembourg

Ward GM, Johnson JE 1986 Validity of the term transfer coefficient. Health Phys 50:411–414

DISCUSSION

Konoplev: One of the problems with using the transfer factor is that it has a high variability. Desmet et al (1991) reported that the soil solution transfer factor for caesium should have a much lower variability. However, the problem with this is how to transfer from the soil solution transfer factor to the aggregated transfer factor. Have you managed to solve this problem?

Howard: No. Many radioecologists have now accepted the premise that the soil solution is important. To estimate bioavailability, scientists have carried out sequential extractions of soil to give them an estimate of what is contained in the water-soluble or ammonium-soluble fraction. However, most have not directly compared the result of sequential extraction with plant uptake. Therefore, many people are making the assumption that their extraction fractions are a direct estimate of what is taken up by the plant. Few people have tested whether the changes they observe with time in the available fraction in the soil are reflected in the amount in the plant. Until we obtain this information and show such correlations it is difficult to translate what we know from conceptual theories into something that we can use at a practical level.

Frissel: Agriculturists have tried to solve the problem of the availability of nutrients in a soil for many years. In the beginning they tried to do this by extraction techniques, just as radioecologists do today, but they failed and therefore had to follow another approach. Basically, they use experimental fields, to which they apply various amounts of fertilizers whilst following the response of the system by observing growth, as well as the quality and quantity of the yield. At the same time, they apply various extraction techniques to the soils of their experimental fields, and they then determine by regression analysis which extraction techniques best explain the fertilizer response. The best extraction technique may differ from nutrient to nutrient and may even depend on the region or type of soil. The result is that agriculturists know exactly what kind of fertilizers have to be applied to obtain optimal yields or optimal profits, although they do not claim to have determined the 'plant-available nutrients'.

Radioecologists cannot follow this approach because they do not have sufficient resources (i.e. a large number of experimental fields contaminated with radionuclides) available. Therefore, radioecologists have to use more fundamental ways to estimate the uptake of radionuclides. The collection of soil solutions or the use of a mild extractant are probably the most promising ones. However, they have to bear in mind the agriculturists' experience and to understand that an extraction method will never be able to simulate a root of a plant.

Håkanson: I have participated in several projects on the sequential extraction of suspended materials in water samples from lakes. Our working hypothesis was that the bioavailable fraction was correlated with the dissolved or easily extractable fraction, but we found that this was usually not the case. Therefore, a chemical fractionation procedure does not represent the biologically available fractionation, and it is why many of the people working on lakes have abandoned fractionation.

Whicker: How much food do grouse consume?

Howard: In our experiments we fed grouse 35 g/day. In the field, people have made estimates of 55 g/day. We used this value of 55 g/day in our chapter, since this is more representative of field conditions with higher food intake rates.

Whicker: How did they measure food intake in the field? I ask this because we are interested in using caesium as a scientific tool for estimating bio-energetic requirements.

Howard: The way that the Institute of Terrestrial Ecology (ITE) has measured food intake in the field is to use a technique developed by Bob Mayes at the Macaulay Land Use Research Institute in Scotland, which uses alkanes as a digestive marker (Dove & Mayes 1986) and has been successfully applied to a large number of different species. We have also used slow-release chromium oxide capsules (Laby et al 1984).

Voigt: I would like to add that we have performed a similar experiment in hens, which are comparable in size to grouse. One animal consumed between about 80–120 g/day (Voigt et al 1993).

Streffer: Have you estimated the dose received by the grouse, not only via food intake but also by external irradiation?

Howard: I can't answer your question about external irradiation. In Scotland, values up to 6000 Bq/kg were measured in grouse after the Chernobyl accident, but these data cannot be compared with external doses for these animals.

Frissel: It has been suggested that caesium uptake by fungal mycelia is time dependent because some species take up caesium from the topsoil and others from the subsoil, and with time caesium moves downwards from the topsoil to the subsoil.

Howard: This is probably correct. It has been shown that there are relationships between mycelium depth, radiocaesium location in the soil profile and contamination levels in fruit bodies.

Frissel: You also remarked that many people believe that almost all of the caesium in the soil is located in the fungal mycelia. This is in agreement with Japanese studies which showed that the transfer factor of stable caesium is equal to the transfer factor of radioactive caesium. This suggests that mushrooms take up both the stable and radioactive forms of caesium.

Howard: The importance of fungal mycelia in radiocaesium soil profiles is currently an interesting hypothesis. More work is required to look at this and also the importance of caesium retention by fungi in the top soil.

Paretzke: K. Bunzl from the GSF Institute für Strahlenschutz has shown that if fungi and weeds are present in the upper soil layer then there is almost no leaching of caesium into deeper soil layers because all the caesium remains bound to these biomaterials at the surface. This is consistent with the remark made by Martin Frissel.

Streffer: Why are different levels of radiocaesium present in different species of mushrooms? What are the mechanisms involved in this differential uptake of radiocaesium into the fungal mycelia?

Howard: There are often differences of up to two or three orders of magnitude between the different species. However, even before the Chernobyl accident, there were high concentrations of radiocaesium (in the order of thousands of Bq per kg) in mushrooms as a result of nuclear weapons testing. We have a lot of information about the levels in species from different countries, so that we can categorize species into low, medium and high accumulators, for instance. There are large differences within species as well as between species, and some of these differences can be accounted for by differences in soil type. However, in answer to your question, the mechanism by which radiocaesium is taken up into the cells will be explained by Gadd (1997, this volume), but it is still not clear why some species are more effective at doing this than others. Olsen (1996) has done some uptake experiments in which he has grown different fungi in different concentrations of potassium. He has shown that, in the presence of low concentrations of potassium, if radiocaesium is added all of the species take up the radiocaesium immediately. When he increases the levels of potassium, however, he starts to observe differences in radiocaesium uptake between the species, suggesting that there is an interaction between potassium and radiocaesium. At the moment we do not understand the physiological reasons for these differences.

Gadd: The uptake of radiocaesium into the hyphae is probably dependent on the external conditions including soil type, pH and caesium concentration. Transport into the cells is generally achieved by a potassium transport system, and translocation of caesium could then occur from the hyphae to the fruiting bodies (see Gadd 1992).

The reports of caesium retention by fungi seem to contradict the data from the grouse. Some mycorrhizae can prevent the transport of toxic metals to aerial plant parts, but it seems that they're not doing that effectively in the case of caesium. This may be explained by its higher mobility in biological systems. Is anything known about this?

Howard: There have only been a few studies on the influences of mycorrhizae on the uptake of radiocaesium, so it is not possible to answer your question definitively. Experiments at the ITE didn't show an increased uptake by mycorrhizal plants compared to non-mycorrhizal plants (Clint & Dighton 1992).

Roed: If the concentration of radiocaesium within the root system is higher than in the soil solution surrounding the roots, doesn't this suggest that an active process is involved?

Frissel: Probably. However, a plant placed in a soil will take up potassium up to a certain level because the potassium content in a plant is homeostatically controlled, i.e. the concentration in the plant does not depend on the concentration in the soil. Caesium behaves similarly to potassium, and therefore it is, in principle, possible to use the Cs/K ratio of the soil to estimate the Cs/K ratio in the plant. By taking into account some discrimination between caesium and potassium, the caesium content in the plant can be estimated by the simple relation:

$$Cs_{plant} = Cs_{soil}/K_{soil}*K_{plant}$$

where * represents the discrimination factor. However, models based on this principle have failed.

Another hypothesis assumes that the uptake can be described by a so-called 'transfer factor', i.e. the ratio between caesium in the plant and caesium in the soil. In this case the uptake is assumed to be independent of the potassium concentration in the soil, and this latter hypothesis is generally accepted. The first hypothesis assumes an active uptake mechanism of caesium, whereas the second does not. The first hypothesis is, from a plant physiological point of view, more attractive, but data seem to favour the second hypothesis. Therefore, there is no hard evidence that an active mechanism of caesium uptake by plant roots exists.

Streffer: Mammalian cells have different active transport systems for potassium and sodium. Therefore, there are good reasons for possible differences between the transport of potassium and caesium. There are differences in the concentrations of caesium in embryos/fetuses and mothers, suggesting that there is a caesium active transport system in mammals. The same could be true for plants.

Gadd: The active transport of caesium via potassium systems has been demonstrated in all groups of micro-organisms including cyanobacteria, bacteria, algae and fungi. All the uptake systems are highly dependent on the concentration of potassium, although we have even found some micro-organisms, for example certain cyanobacteria, that apparently exhibit a higher affinity for caesium under some conditions than for potassium (Avery et al 1991). We have also found some micro-organisms, e.g. the microalga *Chlorella salina*, in which a high concentration of sodium stimulates caesium uptake (Avery et al 1993).

Paretzke: Could this have something to do with the hydration shell of the caesium atom? Caesium has probably got a smaller hydration shell than sodium and potassium.

Gadd: In general terms, although a common behaviour of caesium and potassium may be observed in some systems, there are several cases where potassium and caesium can show markedly different effects. This does not only apply to transport but also to the activation of key metabolic enzymes. For example, if caesium substitutes for potassium, in a potassium-regulated enzyme such as pyruvate kinase the enzyme may be rendered inactive, even though the difference in ionic radius is relatively small between potassium and caesium (Hughes 1987, Perkins & Gadd 1996).

Aarkrog: I would like to make a general comment on semi-natural ecosystems. In a joint Nordic radioecological study carried out after the Chernobyl accident we observed that the contribution of ^{137}Cs from semi-natural ecosystems to the average dietary intake of ^{137}Cs was substantial. There were, however, serious discrepancies between the estimates of these ^{137}Cs intakes. Estimates based on dietary measurements are extremely variable because of the difficulties in determining how many mushrooms, for example, are consumed per year. Our knowledge about the exact food intakes in semi-natural ecosystems is poor.

Howard: I agree. And it's just as important to focus on diet as on the transfer mechanisms if we want to calculate the contribution of different foodstuffs to ingestion dose.

Paretzke: Michael Balonov, could you please give us some information about the total doses received by people living in the highly contaminated areas through semi-natural pathways, such as by eating game and mushrooms, for example?

Balonov: Immediately following the Chernobyl accident there was a high level of transport to milk, which was the main contributor of the internal dose. This transport factor decreased with time— it has a half-life of about one to two years.

Paretzke: I would just like to clarify that your transfer parameter is different from Gabi Voigt's. You have calculated the transfer of the contamination per m^2 into milk, whereas she used the ratio of milk activity to grass activity (Bq/l per Bq/kg).

Balonov: In contrast to the milk contamination, the concentration of radiocaesium in mushrooms and other natural food products such as forest berries and game meat does not decrease rapidly, so that now, 10 years after the accident, semi-natural ecosystems are important contributors to the internal dose, which is about 30–70% in some areas. The total exposure depends on the dominating soil in the area. In the Bryansk area of Russia there is an equal contribution from internal and external doses to the total dose.

Paretzke: What was the total dose received in 1996 through eating products derived from semi-natural ecosystems?

Balonov: In areas that are heavily contaminated as a result of the Chernobyl accident, the total dose is about 1–2 mSv/year, of which about 30–70% is derived from products from semi-natural ecosystems.

Howard: On an individual level this percentage could be much higher; for example, in those with a predilection for mushrooms. In the dietary surveys that Michael Balonov and Per Strand's group were involved with it reached 90–95% (Strand et al 1996).

Paretzke: This is not the case in Germany. According to our experience, some people claim that they eat lots of mushrooms in areas where mushrooms are contaminated by about 3000 Bq/kg, but their measured whole-body radiocaesium content remains within the normal variation (i.e. less than 20 Bq/kg). Also, large amounts of mushrooms are not readily available in winter, at least in Germany, so one should observe a decrease in radiocaesium levels during this season. This is not apparent in your data.

Balonov: I disagree. People from three different areas of Belarus, Russia and Ukraine have a caesium total-body content that is two- to threefold less in spring than in autumn. According to our dietary surveys, the average mushroom consumption is about 10 kg/year per adult person in rural areas of Russia. About 70% of this population collect and consume mushrooms.

Howard: I agree. People in these areas are subsistence farmers: they grow, collect and store whatever food they can.

Voigt: Countermeasures, such as methods of food processing, also have some effect on the levels of radiocaesium in mushrooms.

Håkanson: Radiocaesium is removed effectively from mushrooms by boiling in salted water. Also, stirring helps to reduce the amount of time it takes to remove the radiocaesium, so that many of the vitamins remain.

Howard: Many of the people in the survey were asked about their application of countermeasures. They said their usual method was to boil the mushrooms, but this didn't hold up when we analysed the results. Therefore, this is a countermeasure which is theoretically possible but is not always used in practice.

Balonov: It's difficult to change the traditional method of cooking mushrooms, which in many rural areas is to salt them and eat them without boiling.

Renn: One of the interesting observations relating to some of the Swedish surveys is that there is a correlation between the degree of worry about nuclear accidents and the consumption of mushrooms. Immediately, one tends to conclude that people who eat more mushrooms have increased levels of concern and worry. However, when they compared this behaviour with the actual mushroom consumption patterns, they found that there was no indication that people with high concern had actually consumed more mushrooms, although they claimed they had done so. An interesting hypothesis to explain this strange phenomenon is to reverse the causal order. People who are worried place additional weight and emphasis on their concern by exaggerating their own consumption. If they appear as being victims, their worry becomes even more justified. Similar results have been found when researchers investigated the effects of fishery advisories in contaminated lakes. Residents claimed to eat more fish than they actually did to underline their concern and to initiate more governmental actions towards clear-up. Psychologists call this the victim syndrome, i.e. that somebody who fears being a victim wants to be acknowledged as one.

References

Avery SV, Codd GA, Gadd GM 1991 Caesium accumulation and interactions with other monovalent cations in the cyanobacterium *Synechocystis* PCC 6803. J Gen Microbiol 137:405–413

Avery SV, Codd GA, Gadd GM 1993 Salt stimulation of caesium accumulation by *Chlorella salina*: potential relevance to the development of a biological Cs-removal process. J Gen Microbiol 139:2239–2244

Clint GM, Dighton J 1992 Uptake and accumulation of radiocaesium by mycorrhizal and non-mycorrhizal heather plants. New Phytologist 121:555–561

Desmet GM, Van Loon LR, Howard BJ 1991 Chemical speciation and bioavailability of elements in the environments and their relevance to radioecology. Sci Total Environ 100:105–124

Dove H, Mayes RW 1991 The use of plant wax alkanes as marker substances in studies of the nutrition of herbivores: a review. Aust J Agric Res 42:913–952

Gadd GM 1992 Microbial control of heavy metal pollution. In: Fry JC, Gadd GM, Herbert RA, Jones CW, Watson-Craik I (eds) Microbial control of pollution. Cambridge University Press, Cambridge, p 59–88

Gadd GM 1997 Roles of micro-organisms in the environmental fate of radionuclides. In: Health impacts of large releases of radionuclides. Wiley, Chichester (Ciba Found Symp 203) p 94–108

Hughes MN 1987 Co-ordination compounds in biology. In: Wilkinson G, Gillard RD, McCleverty J (eds) Comprehensive coordination chemistry, vol 6. Pergamon Press, Oxford, p 541–754

Laby RH, Grahan CA, Edwards SR, Kautzner B 1984 A controlled release intrauminal device for the administration of faecal dry-matter markers to the grazing ruminant. Can J Anim Sci 64:337–338

Olsen R 1996 Final/preliminary report for the project 'Radionuclides in fungi in the period 1992–1995'. In: Research programme on radioactive fallout 1992–1995. The Research Council of Norway, Oslo

Perkins J, Gadd GM 1996 Interactions of Cs^+ and other monovalent cations (Li^+, Na^+, Rb^+, NH_4^+) with K^+-dependent pyruvate kinase and malate dehydrogenase from the yeasts *Rhodotorula rubra* and *Saccharomyces cerevisiae*. Mycol Res 100:449–454

Strand P, Howard BJ, Averin V 1996 Transfer of radionuclides to animals, their comparative importance under different agricultural ecosystems and appropriate countermeasures. Experimental collaboration project no. 9: final report. International scientific collaboration on the consequences of the Chernobyl accident (1991–1995). European Commission, Belarus, the Russian Federation, Ukraine. EUR 16539EN. European Commission, Luxembourg

Voigt G, Müller H, Paretzke HG, Bauer T, Röhrmoser G 1993 ^{137}Cs transfer after Chernobyl from fodder into chicken meat and eggs. Health Phys 65:141–146

General discussion I

Konoplev: I would like to talk briefly about the release of so-called 'fuel particles' in the environment during the Chernobyl accident. Radioecologists hardly ever encountered such fuel particles before the accident at Chernobyl. Radioactive particles can be divided into fuel particles, which are uranium oxide particles, and condensation particles, which are produced due to condensation of initially evaporated radionuclides on inert particles. There are many differences in the composition and properties of these two types of particles, and therefore between their behaviours in the environment. The fuel particles contain the complete spectrum of radionuclides. They are almost completely insoluble in water but they can decompose, so that additional amounts of radionuclides can transfer to the soil solution and become available.

During the atmospheric dispersion following the Chernobyl accident, there was a separation of different particles. The heaviest fuel particles containing plutonium and strontium were deposited mainly inside the 30 km exclusion zone. Caesium, on the other hand, due to its volatility, was distributed globally. During the transport of particles containing radiocaesium through the atmosphere, there was a kind of chromatography effect, in that there was a separation of the different chemical forms of ^{137}Cs. Therefore, there are different chemical forms at different sites within the contaminated area. The most unavailable forms were deposited within the 30 km zone, and the most available forms were transported further away (to western Europe, for example). This is one of the reasons why the transfer factors that determined the bioavailability in western Europe were different to those observed in areas such as the Ukraine, Belarus and Russia. The mobile forms of ^{137}Cs in the 30 km exclusion zone around Chernobyl varied between 20–30%; whereas, these values were 40–60% in the Bryansk region of Russia and as high as 85% in Cumbria (Hilton et al 1992). The bioavailability of ^{137}Cs at these sites was different. This was due partly to environmental conditions, such as the soil properties, and also on the initial conditions in the fallout. The bioavailability and transfer factor of ^{190}Sr increased with time, but that this was not the case for ^{137}Cs because this radionuclide is fixed rapidly (within 10 days or so) and the time-scale of its leaching from fuel particles is several years.

Paretzke: Another important factor is that caesium has a much lower melting point than strontium or plutonium, so that most of the ^{137}Cs was released as vapour from the fuel inside the reactor and then attached to aerosols, whereas much of the strontium and plutonium was ejected as fuel particles during the explosion.

Konoplev: We also have data on the fallout in Chernobyl (Konoplev & Bobovnikova 1990). The Russian meteorological service collected samples of fallout on special plates every day after the accident. The sequential extraction experiments were performed in our institute with the plates collected during April/May 1986, and we found that 26% of ^{137}Cs from Chernobyl was in a bioavailable form, and was incorporated in the condensation particles. The remaining 74% was incorporated into fuel particles and was not initially available. However, there was a leaching of ^{137}Cs as well as other radionuclides from the fuel particles with time.

Paretzke: Where were these plates when they were exposed?

Konoplev: They were in the city of Chernobyl, about 15 km from the reactor.

In my opinion, all of the ^{137}Cs in the soil is bioavailable, but the problem is that when we use sequential extraction procedures we observe an instantaneous ratio between different chemical forms. We have to take into account that the real picture of the transfer processes of chemical forms in soil is dynamic and that one day, one week or one year later it may not necessarily be the same.

Howard: I agree. However, people have extracted the same soil over long periods of time to enable models to be developed of soil-to-plant uptake that take these changes in time into consideration. However, this simple approach has only been done in the last few years, and it's 10 years since the Chernobyl accident. It's odd that we have only just started to do this so late in the day.

References

Hilton J, Cambray RS, Green N 1992 Fractionation of radioactive caesium in airborne particles containing bomb fallout, Chernobyl fallout and atmospheric material from the Sellafield site. J Environ Radioact 15:103–108

Konoplev AV, Bobovnikova TsI 1990 Comparative analysis of chemical forms of long-lived radionuclides and their migration and transformation in the environment following the Kyshtym and Chernobyl accidents. Proceedings of seminar on comparative assessment of the environmental impact of radionuclides released during three major nuclear accidents: Kyshtym, Windscale, Chernobyl. Luxemburg, 1–5 October 1990, CEC, 1:371–396

Transport and processes in freshwater ecosystems

Lars Håkanson

Institute of Earth Sciences, Uppsala University, Norbyvägen 18B, S-75236 Uppsala, Sweden

Abstract. The partition coefficient (K_d) and the water retention rate (RR) are fundamental components of dynamic, mass-balance models, not just for radionuclides in fresh water but also for contaminants in all aquatic ecosystems. K_d may be regarded as an 'entry gate' and RR an 'exit gate'. Uncertainties in K_d and RR cause uncertainties in model predictions. Uncertainties in important rates for processes within ecosystems (such as sedimentation, diffusion, advection, bio-uptake and excretion) cannot be adequately evaluated when uncertainties exist for K_d and RR. Empirical data show that there may be a variation in K_d of two orders of magnitude with environmental factors such as pH. This is important because K_d regulates the amount of radionuclides in dissolved and particulate phases, and hence also pelagic and benthic transport. Pelagic transport is directly linked to the outflow and retention of substances in the water mass, and thus also to concentrations and ecological effects. There are many approaches for sub-models of K_d and RR. Which provide the best predictive power? This chapter gives a brief overview and discussion of the benefits and drawbacks of different alternatives for K_d and RR within the framework of a lake model for radiocaesium.

1997 Health impacts of large releases of radionuclides. Wiley, Chichester (Ciba Foundation Symposium 203) p 46–67

This chapter describes the transport of radiocaesium in lakes (Carlsson 1978, Alberts et al 1979, Whicker et al 1990, Monte et al 1993). Most of the results emanate from the International Atomic Energy Agency's VAMP (VAlidation of Model Predictions) project. The new VAMP model is used, but the model and the data will not be presented in detail because this has been done elsewhere (Håkanson et al 1996a,b, IAEA 1997). The VAMP model is a general, state-of-the-art model based on the most fundamental processes. It has been validated against an extensive data set from seven European lakes, which cover a wide range of characteristics (Table 1). The main objective of the model is to predict two target variables: caesium concentrations in predatory fish (used for human consumption) and in water (used for irrigation, drinking water, etc.).

The aim of this chapter is to analyse, mainly by sensitivity simulations, the importance of the partition coefficient (K_d) and the water retention rate (RR). K_d may be regarded as an 'entry gate' to ecosystem models, and RR as an 'exit gate'.

TABLE 1 Data for the seven lakes used to validate the VAMP (VAlidation of Model Predictions) model

Lake	Altitude[a]	Latitude °N	Lake area (km²)	Mean depth (m)	Catchment (km²)	Precipitation (mm/year)	T (years)	pH	Potassium (mg/l)	Primary productivity[b]
Iso Valkjärvi, Finland	126	61	0.042	3.1	0.168	600	3	5.1	0.4	25
Bracciano, Italy	164	42	57	89.5	91.2	900	137	8.5	40	0.8
Øvre Heimdalsvatn, Norway	1090	61	0.78	4.7	23.4	800	0.17	6.8	0.4	27
IJsselmeer, Holland	0	52	1147	4.3	114700	750	0.41	8.5	7	350
Hillesjön, Sweden	10	61	1.6	1.7	19.2	650	0.36	7.3	3	100
Devoke Water, UK	233	54	0.34	4.0	3.06	1840	0.24	6.5	0.55	—
Esthwaite Water, UK	66	54	1	6.4	14.0	1800	0.19	8.0	0.9	350

Lake	Suspended load (mg/l)	Sedimentation rate (g/m²*yr)	¹³⁷Cs deposition (kBq/m²)	Fish	Maximum concentration of ¹³⁷Cs (Bq/kg ww)
Iso Valkjärvi, Finland	0.5	70	70	Whitefish, perch	11650
Bracciano, Italy	0.5	—	0.9	Whitefish	14
Øvre Heimdalsvatn, Norway	0.3	60	130	Minnow, trout	5250
IJsselmeer, Holland	40	500	2.2	Smelt, roach, perch	21
Hillesjön, Sweden	5	0	100	Roach, perch	4750
Devoke Water, UK	0.5	300	17	Perch, trout	1750
Esthwaite Water, UK	1	700	2	—	—

[a]Metres above sea level.
[b]Carbon, g/m² per year.
From IAEA (1997).

Rates

1	k1/2	pike/perch
2	k1/3	pike/roach
3	k2/4	perch/zooplankton
4	k3/4	roach/zooplankton
5	k4/5	zooplankton/phytoplankton
6	k4/6	zooplankton/algae
7	k5/7	phytoplankton/water
8	k6/7	algae/water
9	k1/8	pike/benthos
10	k2/8	perch/benthos
11	k8/9	benthos/sediments
12	k7/9	water/sediments (sedimentation)
13	k9/7	sediments/water (resuspension)
14	k10/7	sediments/water (diffusion)
15	k10/11	sedimentation to non-active layer
16	k10/12	biotransport to non-active layer
17	k10/13	diffusion to non-active layer
18	k14	catchment load
19	k15	direct lake load
20	k16	river input
21	k17	outflow
22	k18	removal by fishing

Variables

A. Biological

1 Pike weight, length and/or age
2 Perch weight, length and/or age
3 Roach weight, length and/or age
4 Zooplankton; species; stage of development; biomass; season of catch
5 Algae; species; stage of development; biomass; season of catch
6 Phytoplankton; species; stage of development; biomass; season of catch
7 Benthos; species; stage of development; biomass; season of catch

B. Lake parameters

1 Lake size
2 Lake volume
3 Lake water retention time
4 Water discharge to lake
5 Sedimentation
6 Resuspension

C. Important relationships

1 Concentration vs. pike weight, length and/or age in the given lake
2 Concentration vs. perch weight, length and/or age in the given lake
3 Concentration vs. roach weight, length and/or age in the given lake
4 Lake load, temporal variability
5 Foodweb, temporal variability

FIG. 1. Rates and model variables often required in traditional ecosystem models for radiocaesium. Important input data for a dynamic model that predicts radionuclides in predatory fish, such as pike, are shown.

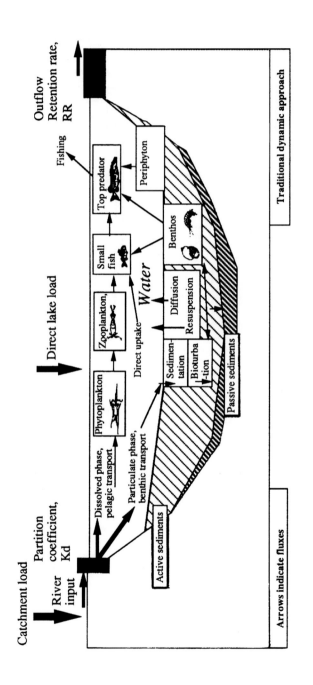

FIG. 2. Compartmental model illustrating the fluxes (arrows, mass per unit time) in a traditional, dynamic model for radiocaesium in a lake ecosystem with compartments (mass units) for top predator, prey fish, zooplankton, phytoplankton, algae, benthos, water and sediments.

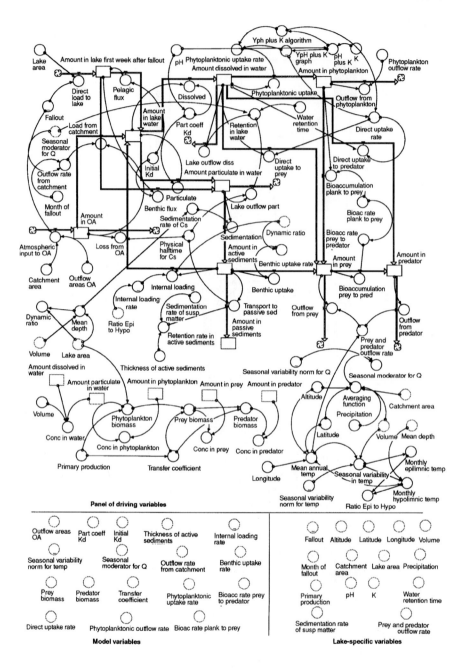

Panel of driving variables

Model variables

Lake-specific variables

Uncertainties in K_d and RR imply that uncertainties for processes within ecosystems, such as sedimentation, diffusion, mixing and bio-uptake, cannot be adequately evaluated. K_d regulates the amount of radionuclides in dissolved and particulate phases and hence pelagic and benthic transport. There are many approaches for sub-models for K_d and RR. Which provide the best predictive power for the targets?

Dynamic models — the VAMP model

Dynamic models are used to quantify fluxes (Vemuri 1978, Jørgensen & Johnsen 1989). Figure 1 lists 22 rates and 18 variables generally used in dynamic models, such as the one outlined in Fig. 2. To make good predictions, one needs reliable estimates of all these rates and variables.

Figure 3 gives an outline of the VAMP model. The environmental variables must be changed for every lake, but the model variables should not be changed. One way to validate models is to regress empirical data against modelled values. The r^2 value and the slope should be close to unity, and the intercept should be at the origin. One can safely assume that r^2 will not be equally high in all validations. In Fig. 4C, a (hypothetical) model is tested in 15 situations. For each validation, r^2, the slope and the coefficient of variation (CV = SD/MV; SD, standard deviation; MV, mean variable) for the r^2 values can be determined.

A definition of predictive power (PP) (Håkanson & Peters 1995) is:

$$PP = R^2/((1.1 - \text{slope})*\text{CV}) \tag{1}$$

where R^2 is the mean r^2. The higher the value of R^2, the higher the PP. If the slope is less than 1, the influence on PP is given by (1.1 − slope). However, if the slope is greater than 1, the slope is set to 1/slope, and the same factor is used (i.e. 1.1 − 1/slope). If the model has a high PP, the CV should be small. The PP of this particular model is 12, which is a rather high value, considering that $R^2 = 0.80$ and CV = 0.19. However, the mean slope is only 0.35, which is far from 1.0.

Three models for radiocaesium in lakes have been tested to determine the relationship between PP and the model (i.e. optimal) size (IAEA 1997).

(1) A small, mixed model (Håkanson 1991) with three compartments (water, prey and predatory fish), six model variables and five lake-specific variables. The

---

FIG. 3. (*opposite*) The VAMP (VAlidation of Model Predictions) model for radiocaesium in lakes. Sub-models for biomass and the seasonal moderators for water discharge (Q) and temperature, and the panel of driving variables are shown. This panel is divided into two parts: model variables and lake-specific variables. The lake-specific or environmental variables change for every lake, but ideally the model variables do not change, unless there are strong reasons to do so. This conservative rigour concerning *ad hoc* adjustments minimizes the 'art' and maximizes the science in building predictive models. From Håkanson et al (1996a).

A

	Model variables $n1$	Lake-specific variables $n2$	$n= n1+n2$	R^2	CV	Slope, MV	1.1-a	PP
Mixed model	6	5	11	0.84	0.66	1.38	0.38	3.39
VAMP model	21	13	34	0.80	0.11	0.77	0.33	21.73
Generic model	29	10	39	0.69	0.41	1.19	0.26	6.48
Empl vs Emp2				0.87	0.09	1.06	0.16	61.73

B

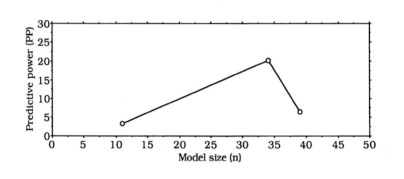

C

Test number	r^2	slope a	if slope >1 then 1/slope	1,1-a
1	0.95	0.90		0.20
2	0.82	0.85		0.25
3	0.77	2.10	0.48	0.62
4	0.96	1.50	0.67	0.43
5	0.66	1.20	0.83	0.27
6	0.55	1.00	1.00	0.10
7	0.88	1.30	0.77	0.33
8	0.46	0.60		0.50
9	0.92	0.80		0.30
10	0.91	1.50	0.67	0.43
11	0.68	1.20	0.83	0.27
12	0.86	2.00	0.50	0.60
13	0.88	0.95		0.15
14	0.92	0.67		0.43
15	0.79	0.80		0.30
MV (=R^2)	**0.80**			**0.35**
SD	0.15			
CV	**0.19**			

Predictive power, PP=0.80/(0.35*0.19)=12.0

PP=R^2/((1,1-slope)*CV)

total number of driving variables (n) is 11. Catchment area, sediments, foodweb and K_d are not represented in this model.

(2) The VAMP model, which is presented in Fig. 3. It has 10 compartments, 21 model variables and 13 lake-specific variables. $n = 34$.

(3) The generic model, which is a traditional model (such as the one illustrated in Fig. 2) with nine compartments, 29 model variables and 10 lake-specific variables. $n = 39$.

These models have been tested using the data for the VAMP lakes. Before comparing empirical data to modelled values, it seems appropriate to discuss uncertainties in the empirical data. Generally, one has access to only limited data. The uncertainty of data series can be tested by a method where one compares two data sets, Emp1 and Emp2, which ideally should be identical. All the data from the first half of the year subsequent to the Chernobyl accident (up to September 1986) are excluded here because during that time conditions were the most variable.

Table 2 shows the r^2 values (Emp1 and Emp2), slopes, PP and n for the available water and fish data sets. All series yielding a PP of less than 1.5 are uncertain and have been omitted, as have cases where $n < 4$. In addition, all the data from Bracciano have been omitted, because this lake contains a significant amount of caesium as a result of weapons testing. Therefore, eight series with acceptable data remain.

The results are summarized in Fig. 4A,B. The smallest model, i.e. the mixed model, yields the lowest PP value; whereas the largest model yields the next lowest PP value. In this case, one obtains, as expected, the highest values of PP when the two empirical data sets are compared (61.73 versus 21.73 for the VAMP model). The smallest model is too small, and the largest model is too large. For every target variable (y) to be predicted there is an optimal size for the predictive model. This size is, however, different for different targets. These validations show that the VAMP model provides good predictions.

Partition coefficients

There are two reasons to focus on K_d. First, K_d plays a fundamental role in dynamic models because a vital requirement is to differentiate between amounts in dissolved and particulate phases. Second, any subsequent prediction depends on the selected K_d.

There are several ways to define K_d. The dissolved phase is generally the fraction that passes through a 0.4–0.45 μm filter; and the particulate phase is the remaining fraction (Haapala 1991). The term 'dissolved' is not equivalent to the bioavailable fraction. The most common expressions for K_d are: $K_d = P/D$ and $K_d = D/(D+P)$, where P is the

---

FIG. 4. Predictive power (PP) for three dynamic models for radiocaesium in lakes. The graph (B) illustrates the relationship between PP and model size (n) for the data given in (A). (C) PP determined from the mean $r^2(R^2)$ mean slope factor and coefficient of variation (CV) for r^2 after 15 (hypothetical) model validations. MV, mean value; SD, standard deviation.

TABLE 2 Comparisons of coefficient of determination (r^2), slope, predictive power (PP) and n for two empirical data sets (Emp1 versus Emp2) for all the available caesium concentrations in water and fish for lakes used to validate the VAMP (VAlidation of Model Predictions) model

Sample	Lake	r^2	Slope	PP[a]	n	Notes[b]
		Emp1 versus Emp2				
Water	IJsselmeer, Holland	0.884	3.020	1.150	4	PP < 1.5
	Iso Valkjärvi, Finland	0.951	0.706	2.414	9	OK
	Devoke Water, UK	0.113	−0.279	0.082	4	PP < 1.5
	Esthwaite Water, UK	0.400	1.247	1.342	8	PP < 1.5
	Hillesjön, Sweden	0.016	0.146	0.017	14	PP < 1.5
	Bracciano[c]	0.986	1.011	11.079	5	'Old Cs'
Whitefish	Iso Valkjärvi, Finland	0.309	0.890	1.471	5	PP < 1.5
	Bracciano, Italy	0.808	0.671	1.883	9	'Old Cs'
Trout	Øvre Heimdalsvatn, Norway	0.862	0.930	5.071	25	OK
	Devoke Water, UK	0.274	0.550	0.498	22	PP < 1.5
Smelt	IJsselmeer, Holland	0.915	0.706	2.322	9	OK
Small perch	Hillesjön, Sweden	0.949	1.171	3.857	5	OK
	Iso Valkjärvi, Finland	0.716	1.351	1.990	12	OK
	IJsselmeer, Holland	0.852	1.804	1.561	9	OK
	Devoke Water, UK	0.017	−0.195	0.013	6	PP < 1.5
Roach	Hillesjön, Sweden	0.653	1.034	9.984	7	OK
Pike	Hillesjön, Sweden	0.854	0.738	2.359	4	OK
	Iso Valkjärvi, Finland	0.440	0.473	0.702	5	PP < 1.5
Large perch	Hillesjön, Sweden	0.867	0.772	2.643	3	$n < 4$
	Devoke Water, UK	0.000	0.009	0.000	9	PP < 1.5

[a]PP = $r^2/(1.1 -$ slope); if slope > 1 then 1/slope.
[b]Empirical data with an acceptable reliability indicated by OK.
[c]Bracciano has still much radiocaesium from old weapons testing. This is not accounted for in these models.

particulate phase and D is the dissolved phase. D/(D+P) gives the fraction of the total (D+P) that appears in dissolved phase.

The value of K_d depends on many factors (Table 3). Salinity and pH influence flocculation, water retention and the settling of suspended particles. Many types of carrier particles exist, such as humus and clays, which have different sizes, shapes, densities and settling velocities (Rancon 1986). The kinetics of the adsorption is often a two-step reaction (Santschi & Honeyman 1989): a fast (within seconds) 'Brownian-pumping' process; followed by a slower (days to weeks) process related

TABLE 3   Published dependencies for the partition coefficient ($K_d = P/D$)

Parameter	Solid	Substance	K_d[a]	Reference[b]
Particulate matter	Natural sediment	Cu, Pb, Cd, Zn, Ni, Hg	—	Balls 1989 (F)
		Al, Fe		Yan et al 1991 (F)
Adsorption time	Natural sediment	Fe, Sn, Cs, Mn, Sb, Be, Zn, Ba, Co, Cd, Se, Hg, Th, Pa	+	Nyffeler et al 1984 (E)
	Faecal pellets	Th, Sn, Pa, Zn, Cs	+	Nyffeler et al 1984 (E)
	Red clay	Fe, Sn Bi, Ce, Co, Mn, Ir	+	Li et al 1984b (E)
		Cd, Sb	0	Li et al 1984b (E)
		Au	—	Li et al 1984b (E)
Desorption time	Red clay	Sn	+	Li et al 1984b (E)
		Ce, Sb, Co, Au, Be, Cd, Mn, Zn, Cs	—	Li et al 1984b (E)
Particulate matter	Red clay	Co, Mn, Zn	+	Li et al 1984b (E)
		Cs	0	Li et al 1984b (E)
		Ce, Hg, Cd, Au, Sb, Ba, Ir, Sb	—	Li et al 1984b (E)
	FeOOH	Co	+	Li et al 1984b (E)
		Zn, Sb	0	Li et al 1984b (E)
		Bi, Ce, Hg, Cd, Au, Mn, Ir	—	Li et al 1984b (E)
	δ-MnO$_2$	Cd, Ba, Zn	+	Li et al 1984b (E)
		Fe, Sn, Bi, Hg, Ce, Au, Cd, Co, Ir, Mn, Sb, Ba	—	Li et al 1984b (E)
	Montmorillonite	Zn	+	Li et al 1984b (E)
		Fe, Sn, Bi, Hg, Ce, Au, Cd, Co, Ir, Mn, Sb, Ba	—	Li et al 1984b (E)
pH	Natural sediment	Zn	+	Tessier et al 1989 (F)
Salinity	Natural sediment	Cd, Cs	—	Turner et al 1993 (F)
		Zn, Mn	+	Turner et al 1993 (F)
pH	Natural sediment, different clays	Be	+	You et al 1989 (E)
Adsorption time	Natural sediment, different clays	Be	+	You et al 1989 (E)
Particulate matter	Natural sediment, different clays	Be	—	You et al 1989 (E)
pH	Natural sediment	Zn, Ni	+	Young et al 1992 (F)
		Cu	0	Young et al 1992 (F)
pH	FeOOH	Cu, Pb, Zn, Cd	+	Balistrieri et al 1983 (E)
Metal concentration	FeOOH	Cu, Pb, Zn, Cd	—	Balistrieri et al 1983 (E)
Salinity	Natural sediment	Bi, Sn, Fe, Hg, Ir	+	Li et al 1984a (E)
		Ce, Co, Mn, Cd, Zn, Cs, Ba, Sb	—	Li et al 1984a (E)

[a]Signs (+, 0, −) indicate responses to an increase in the chemical or physical parameter.
[b](E), experimental measurements; (F), field measurements. (From Johansson & Håkanson 1993).

to aggregation (Nyffeler et al 1984). Adsorption and desorption are also important factors affecting K_d (Li 1984a, You et al 1989).

There are two lake water K_d values in the VAMP model: the 'initial' K_d and the 'regular' K_d. The empirical data for the VAMP lakes indicate that a significant part of the initial fallout was strongly bound to particles, which were quickly deposited on the lake bed. A default assumption in the model is that 50% of the initial fallout directly enters the particulate phase and is then sedimented during the first week after fallout. This fraction subsequently follows either benthic pathways to fish or influences water concentrations via internal loading. The rest will follow pelagic pathways to fish.

The regular K_d differentiates between the particulate and dissolved phases, and it is influenced by pH, i.e. the lower the pH the more ^{137}Cs is in the dissolved phase. This can be quantified by a sub-model. In the future this simple sub-model is likely to be improved and replaced by other approaches accounting for more variables and/or processes. The following sub-model (a dimensionless moderator) is assumed to be valid for lakes with a pH of 4–9. It predicts that 96% of the caesium in the water is in the dissolved phase at pH4, and that this decreases to 26% at pH9. The general formula is:

$$K_d = 1/(x + amp*(pH/bord) - 1)^z \qquad (2)$$

where x and the exponent z are empirical constants, bord is a borderline value (set to pH4), and amp is an amplitude value (calibrated to 1.75). This gives:

$$K_d = 1/(1.04 + (1.75*((pH/4) - 1)^2)) \qquad (3)$$

where K_d is defined here as D/(D+P). This algorithm is based on an ecosystem perspective. It describes mean monthly values for pH and the lake K_d for entire lakes, and not site-specific conditions.

Sensitivity tests have been conducted to determine the significance of the variations and uncertainties in K_d. Figure 5 shows that the model is sensitive to changes in both the initial and the regular K_d. Figures 5A and 5B illustrate how the caesium concentrations in trout and water in Øvre Heimdalsvatn depend on the lake K_d. K_d is first set to 0.53 (default value for pH6.8), followed by 0.36 and then 0.96. Figures 5C and 5D give the corresponding results for the initial K_d, which was set to 0.1, 0.5 (default) and then 0.9.

The choice of K_d value is important for the caesium concentration in fish, but not in water, and there are also great uncertainties in the values. Is the correct value 0.1, 0.5 or 0.9 for the initial K_d? Is equation 3 the most suitable approach for a lake K_d? As long as these uncertainties prevail all other predictions are uncertain.

This model does not include a sediment K_d or factors influencing sediment K_d, such as frayed-edge site concentration, cation exchange capacity of sediment solids, K^+ concentration or NH_4^+ concentration (Cremers et al 1988, Comans & Hockley 1992, De Preter 1990, Hilton 1994).

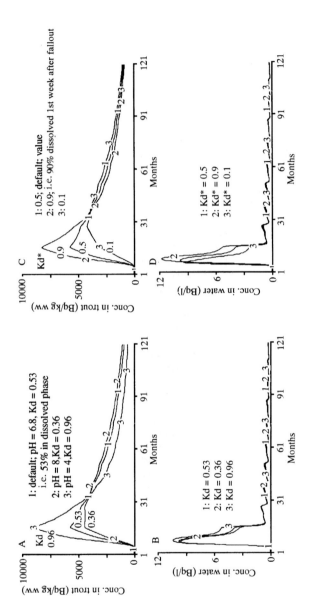

FIG. 5. Sensitivity analyses for K_d in the VAMP (VAlidation of Model Predictions) model using data for Øvre Heimdalsvatn to predict caesium concentration in trout (the top predator in this lake) and lake water. (A) Results for trout and regular lake K_d. (B) Total caesium concentrations in water. (C) Caesium concentrations in trout for initial K_d (K_d^*). (D) Total caesium concentrations in lake water for K_d^*.

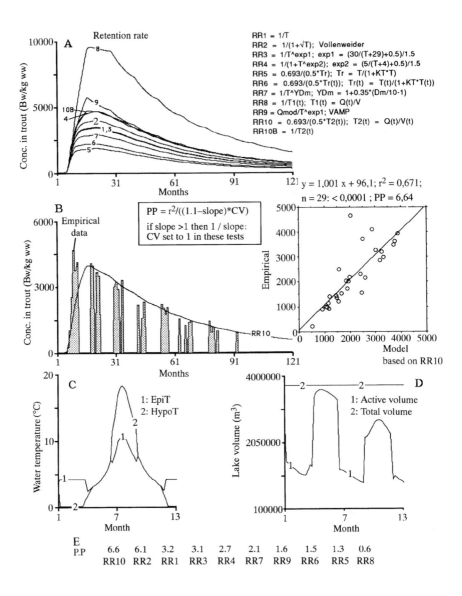

Retention rate

RR1 = 1/T
RR2 = 1/(1+√T); Vollenweider
RR3 = 1/T^exp1; exp1 = (30/(T+29)+0.5)/1.5
RR4 = 1/(1+T^exp2); exp2 = (5/(T+4)+0.5)/1.5
RR5 = 0.693/(0.5*Tr); Tr = T/(1+KT*T)
RR6 = 0.693/(0.5*Tr(t)); Tr(t) = T(t)/(1+KT*T(t))
RR7 = 1/T^YDm; YDm = 1+0.35*(Dm/10-1)
RR8 = 1/T1(t); T1(t) = Q(t)/V
RR9 = Qmod/T^exp1; VAMP
RR10 = 0.693/(0.5*T2(t)); T2(t) = Q(t)/V(t)
RR10B = 1/T2(t)

$y = 1,001 x + 96,1; r^2 = 0,671;$
$n = 29: < 0,0001 ; PP = 6,64$

$PP = r^2/((1.1 - slope)*CV)$

if slope >1 then 1 / slope:
CV set to 1 in these tests

E
P.P   6.6   6.1   3.2   3.1   2.7   2.1   1.6   1.5   1.3   0.6
       RR10 RR2   RR1   RR3   RR4   RR7   RR9   RR6   RR5   RR8

The retention rate

The water retention rate (RR) is generally given by the theoretical water retention time
(T = V/Q) as $1/T$ (i.e. Q/V; where $V =$ volume). Instead of using empirical data on
seasonal variations on tributary discharge, $Q(t)$, which are difficult to access, the
model uses the seasonal moderator for Q (Qmod, which is a dimensionless
expression for seasonal variation in Q [Håkanson & Peters 1995]).

$$RR = Qmod/T \qquad (4)$$

When Qmod has a low value (during the winter), RR is small. In large, stratified lakes
water turnover depends on many processes other than Q (Hutchinson 1957, Simons
1980). Håkanson & Peters (1995) used an approach based on $RR = 1/T^{exp}$. The
exponent (exp) should be about 1 for small, shallow lakes with a T value of about
one month, and it should be less than 1 for lakes with longer T values. The following
algorithm for RR has been derived (IAEA 1997) using the empirical data for the
VAMP lakes:

$$RR = 1/T^{(a/(T+a-1)+b)/(1+b)} \qquad (5)$$

for a = 30 and b = 5. The objective here is to test 10 approaches of the sub-model for RR
(Fig. 6):

(1) the simple physical approach. $RR1 = 1/T$;
(2) a variant of the Vollenweider (1968) approach, $RR2 = 1/(1+T^{0.5})$;
(3) the exponential approach, $RR3 = 1/T^{exp}$, where exp is given by equation 5;
(4) a combination of (2) and (3), $RR4 = 1/(1+T^{exp2})$; where $exp2 = (5/(T+4)+0.5)/$
      1.5, calibrated for best fit for the VAMP lakes;

FIG. 6. (*opposite*) (A) Ten different approaches to define the retention rate (RR) tested within the
framework of the VAMP (VAlidation of Model Predictions) model and to predict caesium
concentrations in trout (top predator) in Øvre Heimdalsvatn. exp, exponent; KT,
sedimentation rate; Q(mod), dimensionless expression for seasonal variations in Q; Q(t),
seasonal variations in tributary discharge; T, theoretical water retention time; Tr,
sedimentation rate for radiocaesium; YDm, dimensionless moderator for mean depth (Dm).
(B) Comparison between empirical data and modelled values using RR10, the corresponding
regression yielding $r^2 = 0.671$ and predictive power (PP) = 6.64 (when the coefficient of
variation [CV] is set to 1). (C) Illustration of predicted epilimnetic (EpiT) and hypolimnetic
(HypoT) temperatures in Øvre Heimdalsvatn. (D) Predicted active volume calculated from
the stratification given in C and related to the total lake volume. (E) Results in terms of a
ranking according to obtained values of PP when all 10 approaches were tested in the same
manner for trout in Øvre Heimdalsvatn as RR10 in B.

(5) the half-life approach, $RR5 = 0.693/(0.5*Tr)$, where $Tr = T/(1+KT*T)$ and KT = the sedimentation rate for radiocaesium (Håkanson & Peters 1995);

(6) the half-life approach using time-dependent T, i.e. $T(t)$, where $RR6 = 0.693/(0.5*Tr(t))$ and $Tr(t) = T(t)/(1+KT*T(t))$;

(7) the mean depth approach, $RR7 = 1/T^{YDm}$, where YDm is a dimensionless moderator for mean depth (Dm) and $YDm = 1+0.35*(Dm/10-1)$ (Håkanson & Peters 1995);

(8) the time-dependent Q approach, where $RR8 = 1/T1(t)$ and $T1(t) = Q(t)/V$;

(9) the VAMP approach (see equations 4 and 5), i.e. $RR9 = Qmod/T^{exp1}$; and

(10) the active volume approach, $RR10 = 0.693/(0.5*T2(t))$, where $T2(t) = Q(t)/V(t)$, or $RR10B = 1/T2(t)$, where $Q(t)$ is measured or predicted water discharge and $V(t)$ is the part of the volume where active transport takes place. The active volume is defined from stratification.

Many of the these approaches are used in modelling in spite of the fact that they are crude and physically unsound. The best approach for ecosystem models should be approach 10. The active volume is determined in three steps:

(1) depth of epilimnetic waters (EpiD in m):
  if $Dmax > 10$ and $Dm > 7.5$, then
  $EpiD = 0 - 7.4*(Strat-1)$ else
  $EpiD = 0 - Dm*(Strat-1)$
  where Dmax = maximum depth in m, Dm = mean depth in m (Dm = V/area), Strat = stratification (see below);

(2) if EpiD <1 m then the active volume (in m³), $V(t)$, is:
  $V(t) = V*((10/(V/Q(t))+9)+0.5)/1.5)$ else
  $V(t) = area*EpiD*((10/(V/Q(t))+9)+0.5)/1.5)$
  where 1 m is an 'initiating' water depth. Operationally, one must decide when stratification starts. Is it more adequate from a modelling perspective, i.e. to achieve maximum PP, to set the initiating water depth to 1 dm, 1 m or to another depth? This approach sets this limit to 1 m, but further studies may improve this;

(3) stratification (Strat, dimensionless). One degree ($+1\,°C$) is added to reduce the amplitude of this ratio for temperatures close to zero:
  if $EpiT > HypoT$ then
  $Strat = (EpiT+1)/(HypoT+1)$ else
  $Strat = (HypoT+1)/(EpiT+1)$.
  The temperatures of surface (EpiT in °C) and bottom (HypoT in °C) water may be measured or predicted by the following method (based on Håkanson & Peters 1995):

(a) during mixing, i.e. if $[EpiT - HypoT] < 6$, then $EpiT = HypoT = (EpiT+HypoT)/2$;

(b) during winter if predicted EpiT <0, then EpiT $= T = 0$, else EpiT; if predicted HypoT $=$ EpiT$/1.75$ <4 then HypoT $= 4$, else HypoT.

During summer and winter stratifications, only the surface water is assumed to take part in mixing and transport. The active volume is much smaller than the entire volume when the lake is stratified (Figs 6C & 6D).

Figure 6B gives the set-up of the tests. Empirical data (trout from Øvre Heinmdalsvatn) are compared to modelled values. In this tests (see Table 4), r^2 is 0.671, the slope is 1.001 and PP (for CV set to 1) is 6.64. These results are valid for RR10. For trout in this lake, RR10 gave the highest PP, and RR8 gave the lowest (Fig. 6E).

An interesting question is: how well does the model behave using different approaches for RR for other lakes? In the following tests (see Table 4), only results for the three best approaches will be given, namely RR10, RR9 and RR2.

From Table 4, one can note several points.

(1) Emp1 corresponds well to Emp2; the highest PP value is 9.89 for roach in Hillesjön, and the lowest value is 1.56 for small perch in IJsselmeer. The mean (MV) PP is 2.80, the standard deviation (SD) among the PP values is 1.23 and the CV is 0.44.

(2) The VAMP model gives almost as good predictions as the empirical data. The highest PP is 5.64 for small perch in Hillesjön, and the lowest PP is 1.04 for small perch in Iso Valkjärvi. The mean PP is 2.24, the SD is 1.45 and the CV is 0.65.

(3) The VAMP model using the modified Vollenweider approach (Voll in Table 4) gives, on average, better predictions than a parallel set of empirical data. The highest PP is 6.1 for trout in Øvre Heimdalsvatn, and the lowest PP is 1.17 for small perch in Iso Valkjärvi. The mean PP is 2.95.

(4) The VAMP model using the active volume approach (Q/V in Table 4) gives the best predictions in terms of the highest mean PP (3.01). The highest PP is 6.7 for trout in Øvre Heimdalsvatn, and the lowest is 1.07 for small perch in Iso Valkjärvi.

(5) If PP is calculated from equation 1, which ought to be relevant for general model comparisons, one can note that Emp1 versus Emp2 yields the highest PP (60.7), the VAMP model with RR2 gives PP $= 47.3$, and RR10 gives PP $= 21$.

These are very promising results.

Conclusions

There are two lake water K_d values in the VAMP model. Great uncertainties exist concerning the proper value for both the initial K_d and for the regular K_d. (Is equation 3 the most relevant algorithm for lake K_d?) As long as these uncertainties concerning the lake K_d values prevail all other predictions are uncertain.

TABLE 4 Comparisons of coefficient of determination (r^2), slope and predictive power (PP) for two empirical data sets (Emp1 versus Emp2). Modelled values according to the original VAluation of Model Predictions (VAMP) model, the VAMP model using the modified Vollenweider approach to express the retention rate (Voll) and the VAMP model with the active volume approach (Q/V) for all available caesium concentrations in water and fish

Sample	Lake	Emp1 versus Emp2			VAMP			Voll			Q/V		
		r^2	slope	PP	r^2	slope	PP	r^2	slope	PP	r^2	slope	PP
Water	Iso Valkjärvi, Finland	0.95	0.71	2.41	0.89	0.65	1.98	0.97	1.33	2.76	0.93	0.83	3.39
Trout	Øvre Heimdalsvatn, Norway	0.86	0.93	5.07	0.66	0.70	1.62	0.77	1.03	6.14	0.67	1.00	6.70
Smelt	IJsselmeer, Holland	0.92	0.71	2.32	0.81	0.75	2.34	0.67	0.64	1.46	0.53	0.67	1.22
Small perch	Hillesjön, Sweden	0.95	1.17	3.86	0.91	1.07	5.64	0.90	1.19	3.52	0.92	1.53	2.05
	Iso Valkjärvi, Finland	0.72	1.35	1.99	0.84	0.30	1.04	0.74	0.47	1.17	0.81	0.34	1.07
	IJsselmeer, Holland	0.85	1.80	1.56	0.77	1.28	2.38	0.68	1.55	1.50	0.62	1.15	2.72
Pike	Hillesjön, Sweden	0.85	0.74	2.36	0.74	0.64	1.58	0.82	0.94	5.17	0.81	0.94	4.94
Roach	Hillesjön, Sweden	0.65	1.03	9.89	0.40	0.81	1.36	0.63	0.76	1.86	0.61	0.79	1.97
	Mean value:	0.87	1.06	2.80	0.80	0.77	2.24	0.79	1.02	2.95	0.75	0.92	3.01
	Standard deviation:	0.08	0.41	1.23	0.09	0.32	1.45	0.11	0.38	1.86	0.15	0.37	1.95
	Coefficient of variation:	0.09	0.39	0.44	0.11	0.41	0.65	0.14	0.37	0.63	0.20	0.41	0.65
	Mean PP:			2.80			2.24			2.95			3.01
	PP from equation 1:			60.68			21.73			47.33			20.97

This work has tested 10 approaches for sub-models for retention rates of lakes. The results indicate that the following three approaches yield the highest PP: the VAMP approach; the modified Vollenweider approach; and the active volume approach. The active volume approach gives promising results. This is encouraging because this is also the causally soundest approach.

It is possible that the active volume approach presented in this chapter may increase the predictive power of different lake models, not only for radiocaesium but also for other substances. However, this remains to be demonstrated. The situation is more problematic with K_d. Much work remains to be done to develop good, validated sub-models for K_d in the case of radionuclides, metals, nutrients and organics in freshwater ecosystems.

Large models are often prescriptive, but not predictive. Large models are simple to build, but difficult to validate. Small size is necessary, but not sufficient, for utility and high PP. Scientific knowledge does not lie in the model alone, nor in the empirical data alone, but in their overlap as validated, predictive models.

Acknowledgements

I thank all my colleagues in the VAMP project (Luigi Monte, John Brittain, Ulla Bergström, Rudic Heling, Vesa Suolanen and Kirsti-Liisa Sjöblom) for constructive co-operation.

References

Alberts JJ, Tilly LJ, Vigerstad TJ 1979 Seasonal cycling of cesium-137 in a reservoir. Science 203:649–651

Carlsson S 1978 A model for the turnover of Cs-137 and potassium in pike (*Esox lucius*). Health Phys 35:549–554

Comans RNJ, Hockley DE 1992 Kinetics of cesium sorption on illite. Geochim Cosmochim Acta 56:1157–1164

Cremers A, Elsen A, De Prater PM, Maes A 1988 Quantitative analysis of radiocaesium in soils. Nature 335:247–249

De Preter P 1990 Radiocesium retention in the aquatic, terrestrial and urban environment: a quantitative and unifying analysis. PhD thesis, Katholieke University, Leuven

Haapala K 1991 Glass fibre and polycarbonate filters for the determination of suspended solids. Vatten 47:226–231

Håkanson L 1991 Ecometric and dynamic modelling: exemplified by cesium in lakes after Chernobyl. Springer-Verlag, Berlin

Håkanson L, Peters RH 1995 Predictive limnology: methods for predictive modelling. SPB Academic Publishing, Amsterdam

Håkanson L, Heling R, Brittain J, Monte L, Bergström U, Suolanen V 1996a Modelling of radiocesium in lakes: the VAMP model. J Environ Radioactivity 33:255–308

Håkanson L, Brittain J, Monte L, Bergström U, Helig R 1996b Modelling of radiocesium in lakes lake sensitivity and remedial strategies. J Environ Radioactivity 33:1–25

Hilton J 1994 Aquatic radioecology post Chernobyl: a review of the past and a look to the future. Manuscript from the Radioecology Seminar, organized by the EU, Lisbon, March 1994

Hutchinson GE 1957 A treatise on limnology. I. Geography, physics, and chemistry. Wiley, New York

IAEA 1997 Models for radiocesium in lakes. Technical document from the VAMP aquatic working group. International Atomic Energy Agency, Vienna

Jørgensen SE, Johnsen J 1989 Principles of environmental science and technology, 2nd edn. Elsevier, Amsterdam (Studies in Environmental Science Series 33)

Li Y-H, Burkhardt L, Buchholtz M, O'Hara P, Santschi PH 1984a Partition of radiotracers between suspended particles and seawater. Geochim Cosmochim Acta 48:2011–2019

Monte L, Fratarcangeli F, Pompei F, Quaggia S, Battella C 1993 Bioaccumulation of Cs-137 in the main species of fishes in lakes of central Italy. Radiochim Acta 60:219–222

Nyffeler UP, Li Y-H, Santschi PH 1984 A kinetic approach to describe trace-element distribution between particles and solution in natural aquatic systems. Geochim Cosmochim Acta 48:1513–1522

Rancon D 1986 Influence of concentration distributions in solid medium on the assessment of radioelement distribution between the liquid and solid phases. In: Sibley TH, Myttenaere C (eds) Application of distribution coefficients to radiological assessment models. Elsevier, Oxon, p 64–71

Santschi PH, Honeyman BD 1989 Radioisotopes as tracers for the interactions between trace metals, colloids and particles in natural waters. In: Vernet J-P (ed) International conference: Heavy metals in the environment, Geneva, September 1989, CEP Consultants, Edinburgh, p 243–252

Simons TJ 1980 Circulation models of lakes and inland seas. Can Bull Fish Aquat Sci 203:1–146

You C-F, Lee T, Li Y-H 1989 The partition of Be between soil and water. Chem Geol 77:105–118

Vemuri V 1978 Modeling of complex systems. Academic Press, Troy, MO

Vollenweider RA 1968 The scientific basis of lake eutrophication, with particular reference to phosphorus and nitrogen as eutrophication factors. Organization for Economic Cooperation and Development, Washington DC

Whicker FW, Pinder JE, Bowling JW, Alberts JJ, Brisbin IL 1990 Distribution of long-lived radionuclides in an abandoned reactor cooling reservoir. Ecol Monogr 60:471–496

DISCUSSION

Streffer: Could you please explain the term K_d?

Håkanson: K_d is the partition coefficient. The total fallout is split into two parts: the soluble phase, which is involved in pelagic transport; and the particulate phase, which will be sedimented and involved in benthic transport. Therefore, the two phases are involved in two different transport processes.

Whicker: When you refer to the 'entry gate' K_d, I presume you're referring to the suspended particulate material, rather than the sediment, versus the dissolved material?

Håkanson: Yes.

Voigt: You showed that there were extreme differences in different types of lakes. Is it possible to use the model that you have developed to describe processes in every lake? For example, we have investigated a lake within a chain of lakes in Bavaria in which there is no stratification (Harladier & Voight 1994). Could your model be applied to such a lake?

Håkanson: Yes, it is a general model. If the lake is not dimictic and there is no stratification, the retention rate is simply 1/T (where T represents the theoretical water retention time).

Renn: Can you clarify the correlation between the two empirical sets. Is it based on the assumption that the measured effects are not governed by stochastic processes? If the measured phenomena are expected to contain stochastic variations, then two different measurements of empirical data that show similar results would not demonstrate high reliability. How do you justify your procedure of comparing two samples if stochastic effects are present?

Håkanson: If one were to measure the radiocaesium concentrations in different pike in the same lake, for example, one would obtain different values. The model is used to predict the mean value and the confidence interval around the mean. This can be achieved in several ways. One way is to divide the measurements into two and take the means of each group. Then two empirical data sets are obtained, which should ideally have the same means. However, if they are not the same, then this gives a measure of the spread, which can be used in uncertainty simulations. This is also how empirical data are compared to model data, and how the model may be validated.

Renn: Is the assumption that the two means have the same value?

Håkanson: The means are supposed to be identical.

Frissel: Is there a relationship between the K_d in soils and the K_d in lakes? I'm asking this because determining the K_d in soils is difficult as it is necessary to use soil : water ratios that are much higher than those that exist in the soil. In lakes this problem is unlikely to exist.

Håkanson: The lake K_d is probably based on different driving variables than the soil K_d, but it may be possible to use the same general approach to develop a model for soil K_d.

Frissel: What type of driving variables are you referring to?

Håkanson: Alexei Konoplev can give you some examples because he is an expert in this field.

Konoplev: The K_d is a key parameter in almost all radioecological models, including aquatic, terrestrial, terrestrial/aquatic interface and soil-to-plant transport models. However, the uncertainty of the total K_d value can be relatively high; for example, the K_d value for radiocaesium can range between four orders of magnitude. However, if one considers the physico-chemical processes that are responsible for caesium distribution, this variability can be explained in terms of the absorption characteristics and fixation potential of the corresponding solid. We have demonstrated that the so-called 'exchangeable' K_d value, which is normalized to the available forms of radiocaesium in the soil, is much less variable. Another advantage of the exchangeable K_d is that, in contrast to the total K_d value, it is not time dependent. The total K_d is used in most of the radioecological models, so the only problem remaining is to replace the total K_d with the exchangeable K_d for each specific time period, which requires some experimental knowledge or predictions of the fixation rates and remobilization rates.

Voigt: Is the remobilization of radionuclides from sediments into water considered in your model?

Håkanson: Yes. We generally divide the sediments into two parts: those that are affected by active processes and the bio-passive sediments. We account for retention rates, diffusion rates and sedimentation rates. The age of the active sediments is also important because it regulates the retention rate of radiocaesium in the active sediment layer.

Voigt: We have found that these rates can vary between lakes.

Whicker: We're trying to gather some data on K_d in reservoir sediments at the Savannah River Site in South Carolina, USA. We have measured a K_d that achieves equilibrium fairly rapidly. However, I have a gut feeling that what we really need to be measuring to make these models work well are the adsorption and desorption rate constants because the time-scales will be critical, particularly if there is a high water turnover rate in the lake. What would you advise us to do? Should we be measuring these constants in addition the equilibrium K_d?

Håkanson: Could you first describe your experiments?

Whicker: If we follow a batch equilibrium method, where we add ^{134}Cs to a slurry and observe a decrease in water, we find that an apparent equilibrium is reached within a few days and the K_d can be calculated. However, the equilibrium changes slowly, but significantly, over the following two months or so. We have also found that the equilibrium is affected by pH and the sediment-to-water slurry ratio. Are we on the right track?

Håkanson: Yes, because there are data which indicate that the absorption process is a two-step process, i.e. there is an initial step, which is rapid, followed by a more prolonged and slower step.

Whicker: We're also doing these experiments simultaneously with ^{85}Sr, which reaches an equilibrium quickly and behaves like a simple two-compartment exchange.

Konoplev: I support what you are saying because the K_d value is dynamic, and therefore kinetic processes must be taken into account. Moreover, in the field there is an interaction between physico-chemical processes and hydrological processes. It is possible that in some hydrological systems an equilibrium is never reached, so that we have to work with non-equilibrium conditions.

Håkanson: In my opinion, even if we develop a good mechanistic model for soil K_d many uncertainties would remain. However, the development of such a model would still be a major step forward. The development of these predicted models for K_d is a scientific challenge.

Paretzke: Models should be as complex as necessary. The concept of K_d is simple but it doesn't give the whole truth, and it is therefore necessary to incorporate other variables. As long as one does this carefully, the resulting complex model can actually be much simpler and accurate to apply in the long run.

Roed: However, sometimes it may be more useful to start off with a simple model, even though it may have many uncertainties.

Frissel: Would it be possible to predict the K_d as a function of the pH and redox potential? The redox potential determines to a large extent the absorbing surface; for example, at a low redox potential many aluminium and iron oxides go into solution and consequently the absorbing surfaces disappear.

Håkanson: The redox potential is easy to measure and it is probably a good predictor of lake K_d. However, it is still necessary to measure the amount of suspended material, and perhaps also ammonium, pH, potassium and the amount of coloured substances. These are five readily accessible driving variables, and a model based on all of them would be useful in determining lake K_d.

Balonov: Do you use a formal procedure for categorizing the number of variables?

Håkanson: When we define the model we start off with a panel of driving variables, and then we divide them into lake-specific variables, which are changed for each lake, and model variables which are preferably not changed. This division is only the first step at trying to minimize the element of 'art' in modelling.

Reference

Harladier R, Voigt G 1994 Distribution of radiocaesium activities in the waters of a Bavarian chain of lakes. Radiat Environ Biophys 33:365–372

Radioactive contamination of the marine environment

A. Aarkrog[1]

Environmental Science and Technology Department MIL-114, Risø National Laboratory, PO Box 49, DK-4000 Roskilde, Denmark

More than 70% of the earth is covered with oceans. These have a mean depth of 4 km and, as the surface area of the earth is 510 million km^2, the total volume of the oceans is approximately 10^{21} l. Therefore, they are by far the most important source of water on the earth. The capacity of the oceans is enormous. For instance, if the total amount of man-made radioactivity was diluted in the oceans, one would still not end up with an amount that is comparable to the naturally occurring radioactivity in the oceans.

The major source of man-made radioactivity in the oceans is derived from nuclear weapons testing fallout, which occurred mostly in the late 1950s and early 1960s. For example, 0.9 EBq of ^{137}Cs and 0.6 EBq of ^{90}Sr were introduced in this way. Only 60% of the released activity was disposed of in the oceans, rather than 70%, because the nuclear weapons testing occurred mainly in the Northern hemisphere, and the land masses cover more of the Northern hemisphere than the Southern hemisphere.

There have also been other releases into the oceans; for example, the water-borne discharges from the Sellafield reprocessing plant in the UK, which occurred from the mid-1970s to the mid-1980s. During this decade, in the order of 40 PBq of ^{137}Cs was discharged into the Irish sea, and from there it was transported into the north Atlantic ocean.

The third important source of radioactivity was the Chernobyl accident. Although most of this radioactivity was distributed over the land masses, about 5 PBq was deposited into the Baltic Sea and about 3 PBq into the Black Sea. The radioactive debris from Chernobyl was distributed around the Northern hemisphere, so some of the radioactivity must have been deposited in the North Atlantic ocean. We have estimated that about 5–10 PBq ^{137}Cs was deposited in oceans more distant than the

---

[1]Unfortunately, due to illness, Per Strand could not give the scheduled presentation on this subject. However, Asker Aarkrog kindly stepped in at short notice and gave this general introduction to the discussion.

Baltic or Black Seas. Hence, about 10–20% of the total release of ^{137}Cs from the Chernobyl accident was disposed of into the oceans.

There have also been a number of local contaminations of the oceans. Among these, I would like to mention satellite failures. For example, the SNAP-9A satellite, which burned up over the South Atlantic ocean in the early 1960s, became a major source of ^{238}Pu pollution. This is the reason why there is an increased ^{238}Pu : ^{239}Pu ratio, mostly in the Southern hemisphere, in global fallout. There have also been two Cosmos satellite failures — one Russian satellite, Cosmos 954, burned up over Canada and the other landed in the Indian ocean — but there have been no reports of measurable contamination of the ocean resulting from these failures.

There are also a number of nuclear submarines on the bottom of the sea; for example, the American Thresher submarine in the Atlantic ocean and the Comsomolets submarine in the Norwegian–Barents sea. There has been some concern over the latter submarine, which lies 1700 m deep into the sea and has two nuclear weapons containing about 6 kg of plutonium and a nuclear reactor.

Furthermore, there have been several accidents with nuclear weapons; for example, the Palomares accident in Spain in 1966 and the Thule accident in Greenland in 1968. As a result of these accidents radioactivity reached the marine environment (about 0.5 kg plutonium is present in the marine sediments at Thule), although most of it was recovered.

Finally, nuclear material is also dumped into the sea. We have known for many years about the European dump site, i.e. the Nuclear Energy Agency dump site in the North East Atlantic. Spain and Ireland are the two countries closest to this site. There are also specific dump sites in the Pacific ocean near the USA. The Russians have a dump site at Novaya Zemlya. This was revealed some years ago in the so-called 'white book' by President Yeltsin's environmental advisor Yablokov, who told us about the dumping of nuclear material in the Kara sea, which is close to the Barents sea. In the beginning it was difficult to determine how much material was dumped and what isotopes it contained. However, it's clear that there are six nuclear reactors with spent fuel at the moment. The so-called International Arctic Seas Assessment Project (IASAP) group at the International Atomic Energy Agency (IAEA) in Vienna have reported that the total amount of radioactivity currently present in these reactors is in the order of 5 PBq. Originally, the amount of activity was estimated to be as high as 100 PBq, but this value referred to the amount at the time of dumping. There have been several joint Norwegian–Russian expeditions to the dump site at Novaya Zemlya. They have measured the surrounding areas around these reactors and found that there are enhanced levels of radioactivity near the reactors, although the Kara sea is not significantly contaminated. Furthermore, it has been calculated that if all the activity in these reactors were released into the world's oceans, the total collective dose to humans would be in the order of 10 person-sieverts, which is negligible. Therefore, it's not fair to say that the dumped material at Novaya Zemlya presents a real danger to the environment. There is also another dump site close to Japan, which the Japanese have been concerned about and which is under examination.

There was a remarkable accident in 1987. In Russia a number of lighthouses along the Siberian coast are operated by ^{90}Sr generators, the typical source sizes of which are in the order of 10–15 PBq. Such a source was being carried by a helicopter, which crashed at Sakhalin Island. The source was not recovered; however, the containment of the source was resistant enough to prevent radioactivity from being released into the sea. There would otherwise have been a significant pollution of ^{90}Sr in the local seas.

I would also like to mention that a few years ago there was a group from the IAEA called MARDOS, whose intention was to calculate the collective doses to humans from selected radionuclides in the oceans. Until then the United Nations Scientific Committee on the Effects of Atomic Radiation (UNSCEAR) had only been concerned with terrestrial environments, but they thought it would be helpful to have an indication of the doses received from marine environments. MARDOS chose ^{137}Cs as a representative anthropogenic radionuclide and ^{210}Po for a naturally occurring radionuclide. They estimated the doses for the year 1990 in two ways. First, they measured the radioactivity concentrations in the sea water worldwide, and then determined the doses from the concentration factors given for fish and shellfish in the literature, and from the consumption rates by humans. Second, they measured the radioactivity levels directly in fish and shellfish from all over the world. They found that for ^{137}Cs the two approaches gave the same estimate, namely 160 person-sieverts. This was not the case for ^{210}Po, which was in the order of 30 000 person-sieverts $+/-$ 10 000 person-sieverts. These doses, especially the doses from ^{137}Cs, are small, i.e. two to three orders of magnitude less compared with the dose received from terrestrial food-chains.

DISCUSSION

Paretzke: Can you please say a few words about the activity levels of naturally occurring ^{210}Po in fish. It seems that the data regarding the negligibility of exposures to the marine environment do not hold for naturally occurring ^{210}Po.

Aarkrog: The present dose from naturally occurring ^{210}Po is about 100-fold larger than the dose from all anthropogenic radionuclides in the marine environment. Furthermore, it's true that in the human diet ^{210}Po from the marine environment is a significant contributor to the dose: about 50% of the dose from polonium in the human diet comes from the marine environment, although this is obviously dependent on the amount of fish, and in particular shellfish, consumed.

Paretzke: On the Marshall Islands, if one fish is eaten per day the total yearly dose from ^{210}Po can represent a significant proportion of the total natural exposure.

Aarkrog: It seems that way. The global collective dose has been estimated at about 30 000 person-sieverts, so if that is divided by the 4 billion people exposed in the Northern hemisphere, the average individual dose is about 7 μSv. Of course this is an average, and there are large variations in the amounts of fish and shellfish people consume.

Cigna: I would like to add to this discussion some information about the MARINA Project. It was set up by the Commission of the European Communities in 1985 to look at the radiological impact of radionuclides, both natural and anthropogenic, in northern European marine waters. The major contributors to the collective exposure of the European Community population are naturally occurring radionuclides. The next most significant source is discharges from civil nuclear sites; however, the maximum collective dose rate from this source (330 person-sieverts/year) is around an order of magnitude lower than that from natural marine radioactivity and about three orders of magnitude lower than the collective dose rate to the European Community population from all natural radioactivity including that of terrestrial origin. The collective exposure from weapons testing fallout and the Chernobyl fallout is somewhat less than that from civil nuclear discharges.

The total collective dose delivered to the population of the European Community up to the year 2500 from civil nuclear plants has been estimated as 5300 person-sieverts, approximately 88% of which has been attributed to the Sellafield reprocessing plant (CEC 1990).

A similar exercise (the MARINA-MED Project) was repeated in 1992 with reference to the radioactive materials in the Mediterranean Sea. The total dose delivered to the population of the European Community up to the year 2500 from civil nuclear plants was estimated as 2 person-sieverts, about 80% of which was attributed to the discharges from the French nuclear plants in the Rhone valley (Cigna et al 1994).

Another study, the Co-ordinated Research and Environmental Surveillance Programme (CRESP), was set up by the Nuclear Energy Agency of the Organization for Economic Cooperation and Development (NEA-OECD). It was established in 1980 for an initial period of four years (and subsequently extended in 1985 and 1990 for further five-year periods) with the hope of strengthening the scientific and technical bases of future assessments of the northeastern Atlantic dump site, which have to be carried out according to an OECD council decision establishing a multilateral consultation and surveillance mechanisms for sea dumping of radioactive waste (NEA 1981, 1986, 1990). The first models were rather rough, but they have since been refined and are now closer to reality. The conclusion was that the doses to humans for all these radionuclides are negligible.

Aarkrog: In terms of the dumping of radioactive waste into the sea, although the levels may comply with the International Commission on Radiological Protection's dose limits to humans, it is possible that animals living close to the dump sites could receive doses which are harmful to them. However, the conclusion is that animal populations are not affected by this dumping.

Gadd: You mentioned that the deposition of ^{137}Cs into the vast volumes of the ocean was insignificant because of dilution. Potentially, a different message can be obtained from that kind of statement just as it can be obtained for any other pollutant that finds its way into the sea. It should be clearly understood that many of these pollutants, which also include toxic metals, metals, xenobiotics and other radionuclides, can be distributed from point sources, where there may be severe and accumulative effects on the biota.

Aarkrog: That's a fair statement. When I mentioned this, it was more it the context of dumping waste deep in the oceans, where it's unlikely to affect humans directly. Of course it would be different if radioactivity was discharged in coastal areas. The discharge into the Baltic Sea following the Chernobyl accident is an example of this, although the activity there has now decreased significantly.

Paretzke: What is the effective half-life of ^{137}Cs in the Baltic sea?

Aarkrog: The effective mean residence time of ^{137}Cs in the Baltic sea is around 15 years, because the mean residence time of the water is in the order of 20–25 years.

Paretzke: Is the dilution due to water exchange rather than sedimentation?

Aarkrog: Yes.

Goldman: There were some studies of the deep trench in the Pacific which showed that if radioactive material is deposited at a very deep depths, it mixes extremely slowly, if at all, with the upper ocean layers (Eisenbud 1987).

What is the contribution to the North Arctic oceans from the drainage of the Ob River, which has a high level of contamination from the Mayak plant and from Chelyabinsk reases?

Aarkrog: That's a good question, and I cannot give you an answer. The exact inventories of man-made radioactivity in the Arctic oceans are presently unknown. The inventory of radioactivity in the Arctic ocean has been calculated to be twofold higher than the input into the Arctic ocean from global fallout and other known sources (Sellafield and Chernobyl). At first, we believed that the missing radioactivity came from the run-off from the Russian river systems. However, we are now not so sure because we have measured these river systems and found no strong indication of a substantial release of radioactivity. We then thought that the missing radioactivity could have come from local fallout from the Novaya Zemlya test site. However, our Russian colleagues have told us that there was not much local fallout because the explosions were powerful high altitude shots which injected the radioactive debris into the stratosphere. The Russians also claimed that the input from the Novaya Zemlya nuclear test series to the global fallout situation was threefold less than that estimated by the United Nations Scientific Committee on the Effects of Atomic Radiation (UNSCEAR), so there are many uncertainties.

Håkanson: I have one small comment on these inventories. In the Baltic about 60–80% of all the suspended materials come from land uplift after glaciation, and the suspended materials also vary depending on the character of the coastal area. Generally, the resuspension of deposited material dominates the fluxes of all types of materials and therefore resuspension is extremely important.

References

CEC 1990 The radiological exposure of the population of the European Community from radioactivity in North European marine waters. Project 'MARINA'. Commission of the European Communities, Radiation Protection 47. Report EUR 12483 EN, Luxembourg

Cigna A, Delfanti R, Serro R 1994 The radiological exposure of the population of the European Community to radioactivity in the Mediterranean sea. 'MARINA-MED' Project. Radiation Protection 70. Report EUR 15564 EN, Luxembourg

Eisenbud M 1987 Environmental Radioactivity, 3rd edn. Academic Press, New York, p 111–112

NEA 1981 Research and environmental surveillance programme related to sea disposal of radioactive waste. Nuclear Energy Agency of the Organization for Economic Co-operation and Development, Paris, p 38

NEA 1986 CRESP Activity Report 1981–1985. Nuclear Energy Agency of the Organization for Economic Co-operation and Development, Paris, p 63

NEA 1990 CRESP Activity Report 1986–1990. Nuclear Energy Agency of the Organization for Economic Co-operation and Development, Paris, p 152

Impacts on plant and animal populations

F. Ward Whicker

Department of Radiological Health Sciences, Colorado State University, Fort Collins, CO 80523, USA

Abstract. Historical experiments and observations in radioactively contaminated environments have documented radiation impacts on natural plant communities and animal populations. General findings from these studies are reviewed. Despite much information on the response of individual organisms to radiation in the laboratory, the database is more limited and the interpretations more complex for natural populations and communities exposed to radionuclides. These complications are discussed as they pertain to plants and animals in natural environments. Paradigms concerning the recovery of radiation-damaged communities and ecosystems, and areas of needed research are discussed.

1997 Health impacts of large releases of radionuclides. Wiley, Chichester (Ciba Foundation Symposium 203) p 74–88

Ever since the dawn of the nuclear age, we have lived with the possibility of large releases of radionuclides into the environment, either through accidents or nuclear war. Although nuclear war now seems less likely, there is no certainty that large accidents won't happen again. Even certain 'routine' releases during a portion of the cold war resulted in local and sometimes regional contamination of significance to human health and environmental quality. Although our first concern about radioactive contamination is centred on human health, the plants and animals that form ecosystems upon which all life is dependent are in some ways more vulnerable to radiation impacts than are humans. It was estimated that plants and animals near Chernobyl, for example, experienced doses typically 30–100-fold greater than the doses received by people in the region (Alexakhin 1993). It is therefore important to learn as much as possible about the effects of radioactive contamination on plants and animals, as well as on humans.

Many data have accumulated over the last four decades on the effects of ionizing radiation on plants and animals. However, only a small portion of this information is directly relevant to understanding the responses of plant and animal populations in natural environments. Most research has emphasized individual rather than population responses, mortality rather than reproduction, acute rather than chronic irradiation, and external gamma radiation rather than exposure to individual or mixed radionuclides in the environment. Population and community responses to stress are much more complex than those of individual organisms in the laboratory. In the long run, reproduction is generally a more radiosensitive determinant of population response than is mortality, but one can ask whether there are even more sensitive determinants. Radionuclide contamination involves complex, time- and space-dependent dosimetry, at scales ranging from micrometres to kilometres, which can be unique to each situation. In contaminated environments damage competes with repair, recovery, selective forces determined by the size of the stressed area, and soil, climatic and biological variables. This complexity impedes our full understanding.

Nevertheless, research has provided some general notions and a framework for making broad predictions. Furthermore, observations of actual impacts of large radionuclide releases on plants and animals have strengthened many ideas, but they have also raised new questions. My goals in this chapter are: (1) to summarize some of the more important concepts that have developed from research on natural plant and animal populations; and (2) to suggest questions that need to be answered before we can have confidence in our ability to predict impacts of large radionuclide releases on natural populations.

Historical experiments and observations

Individual species exhibit large differences in their basic sensitivity to ionizing radiation. For example, acute doses to produce a rapid, 100% mortality range from a few Gy for the most sensitive mammals to nearly 10^4 Gy for the most resistant viruses, bacteria and primitive plants (Fig. 1). Within taxonomic groups, there are also wide ranges of sensitivity, particularly among the plants, insects and bacteria. Such variations stem largely from inherent differences in cellular and molecular characteristics. Besides mortality, there are other damage endpoints that occur at lower doses. Some are shown in Fig. 2 for higher plants exposed to chronic radiation (Sparrow & Woodwell 1963). There are also large species variations in these other endpoints.

A result of species differences in radiosensitivity is that the response of biological communities to exposures damaging to some but not all members is confounded by secondary responses. For example, resistant plants might increase in number and vigour using light and nutrients that become available when a dominant, sensitive tree is killed by radiation. Species that were directly or indirectly dependent on the radiosensitive tree might exhibit declines, whether or not they were impacted by radiation. Conversely, species that associate with radioresistant plants might increase in numbers, provided that they can tolerate the radiation stress.

Studies on the effects of ionizing radiation on plants and animals have used several approaches. Early work relied on X-ray machines and fixed gamma sources in laboratory settings. More ecologically relevant work has used large, fixed gamma ray sources in ecosystems (Woodwell 1967, Fraley & Whicker 1973, Alexakhin et al 1994),

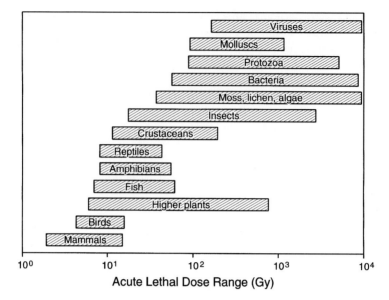

FIG. 1.   Approximate acute dose ranges causing 100% mortality in various taxonomic groups (Whicker & Schultz 1982).

observations near an unshielded reactor (Platt 1965), observations in areas of high natural background radiation (Léonard et al 1985), application of radioactive particles to small ecosystems (Murphy & McCormick 1971) and observations in areas affected by large accidental releases (Kryshev 1992, Tikhomirov & Shcheglov 1994). Some primary observations on the initial impacts of the Chernobyl and Kyshtym accidents are shown in Table 1. A summary of impacts associated with the

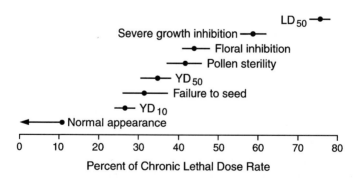

FIG. 2. Per cent of the chronic 100% lethal dose rate that produces other damage endpoints in higher plants (Sparrow & Woodwell 1963). LD_{50}, dose rate producing 50% mortality; YD_n, dose rate producing a growth yield of n% lower than normal.

TABLE 1 Estimated dose ranges absorbed by critical biological tissues within the first 15–60 days after the accidents at Chernobyl and Kyshtym, and some documented effects (Tikhomirov & Shcheglov 1994, Alexakhin 1993, Arkhipov et al 1994, Kryshev 1992, Skuterud et al 1994, Smirnov 1993)

Dose range (Gy)	Impacts on plants	Impacts on animals
<0.1	No visible damage; chromosome damage in spiderwort stamens	Documented impacts not located by author
0.1–0.3	Minor reduction in growth and reproduction in pines; chromosome damage in pines	Impaired reproduction in rodents; chromosomal damage in mice
3–5	Growth inhibition and histological changes in pines	No visible changes in fish populations
5–10	Severe growth reduction, needle damage, morphological change and sterility in pines; threshold for ecosytem-level disruption	Decreased numbers of soil and litter fauna; physiological changes in rodents
10–25	Growth cessation, severe crown damage and insect infestation of pines	Reductions in mouse populations
25–100	Severe mortality in pines; morphological damage, delayed sprouting and early leaf fall in deciduous trees; significant ecosystem-level disruption	Mortality of juvenile invertebrates
>100	Complete mortality in pines; severe crown damage in deciduous trees	Documented impacts not located by author
>200	Lethality of deciduous trees	Acute lethality in rodents
>700	Damage to herbaceous communities	Documented impacts not located by author

more consistent chronic doses 1–1.5 years after the Kyshtym accident (Table 2) was prepared by J. R. Trabalka (Barnthouse 1995).

Effects on plants and plant communities

An example of the effects of radionuclides on a dominant yet radiosensitive species is the pine forest near the Chernobyl nuclear power plant. It was known long before the accident in 1986 that most coniferous trees (e.g. pines, spruces and firs) were relatively sensitive to ionizing radiation. The experiments of Sparrow, Woodwell and others showed that short-term doses of only 1 Gy could slightly damage, and those over 20 Gy could devastate coniferous forests (Whicker & Fraley 1974). Coniferous forests are the most radiosensitive of the major plant communities studied (Table 3). These findings were strengthened by the mortality rates of pines near Chernobyl, and in the

TABLE 2   Estimated ranges of chronic dose rates from 1–1.5 years following the Kyshtym accident, and some documented effects on populations. Based on a review by J. R. Trabalka (Barnthouse 1995)

Dose rate range (Gy/day)	Impacts observed
<0.05	A variety of sublethal effects in pines
0.05–0.1	Complete mortality of pines within two years
>0.2	Reduced nesting of birds
>0.3	Reduced seed production and germination, and morphological changes in leaves of some plants; withered crowns, underdeveloped leaves and phenological shifts in birch trees
>0.5	Complete mortality of birch trees; complete mortality of grasses and forbs, with renewal buds at or near the soil surface
>3	Complete mortality of all higher plants

province of Chelyabinsk as a result of the waste tank explosion at the Mayak facility near Kyshtym in 1957. These studies, summarized by Alexakhin (1993), suggested that annual doses in the order of 5 Gy were required for detectable ecosystem disruption, with somewhat larger doses required for severe damage. So dramatic was the response

TABLE 3   Estimated short-term[a] radiation doses required to damage various plant communities (Whicker & Fraley 1974)

Community type	Doses (Gy) to produce		
	Minor effects[b]	Intermediate effects[c]	Severe effects[d]
Coniferous forest	1–10	10–20	>20
Deciduous forest	10–50	50–100	>100
Shrub	10–50	50–200	>200
Tropical rain forest	40–100	100–400	>400
Rock outcrop (herbaceous)	80–100	100–400	>400
Old fields (herbaceous)[e]	30–100	100–1000	>1000
Grassland	80–100	100–1000	>1000
Moss–lichen	100–500	500–5000	>5000

[a]Short-term doses delivered over eight to 30 days according to the literature on which this table is based. Doses might be reduced by factors of two to four for acute irradiation.
[b]Minor effects include changes in productivity, reproduction and phenology. Recovery occurs rapidly after irradiation.
[c]Intermediate effects include changes in species composition and diversity through selective mortality. Recovery may require from one to several generations.
[d]Severe effects include drastic changes in species composition and mortality of most higher plant species. Recovery may be slow (years to decades or more).
[e]Abandoned agricultural fields.

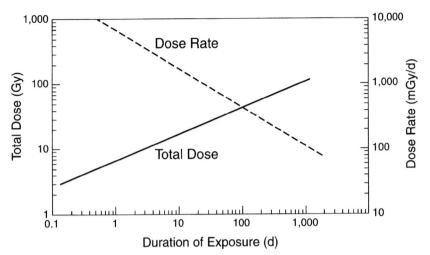

FIG. 3. Relationships between total dose, dose rate and duration of exposure for 50% mortality in pines. Relationships represent several different studies cited in IAEA (1992).

of more than 4 km² of pine forest to the Chernobyl accident, that satellite imagery could be used to observe the progression of damage (McClellan et al 1994).

The interpretation of radiation responses after a release of radionuclides is complicated by several factors. For example, total dose may not be as important as the dose rate and duration of specific dose rates. Data from several experiments were combined to show that for a given endpoint, such as 50% mortality in pines, the total dose required depends on both dose rate and duration of exposure (Fig. 3). A one-day exposure providing 7 Gy has an effect equivalent to a dose of 25 Gy delivered over 30 days, or a dose of 70 Gy delivered over a period of one year. For a mixture of radionuclides from a reactor accident, dose rates decline rapidly with time. For Chernobyl fallout on pine crowns, McClellan et al (1994) estimated that the declining dose rate was roughly comparable to a constant dose rate for a duration of 21 days, during which time about 80% of the actual cumulative dose would be delivered. Clearly, the specific conditions of any accident would affect such calculations. At Kyshtym, for example, the initial rate of decline in dose rate was reduced, due to less short-lived radioactivity in the debris.

Another consideration is the relationship between the accumulated dose and the time required to reach a particular damage endpoint. In general, the greater the initial dose, the more rapid the manifestation of damage. McClellan et al (1994) showed that the short-term (eight to 30 days) doses causing 100 % mortality in pines varied from 40 Gy if lethality were complete within 200 days to 100 Gy if lethality were to occur in 10 days. This relationship, however, depends on whether the plants are actively growing or dormant when exposed. Plants exposed continuously whilst dormant may accumulate damage without obviously showing it until climatic conditions permit active growth (Whicker & Fraley 1974, Tikhomirov & Romanov 1993).

Several generalities have emerged from past research. Molecular and cellular characteristics — such as large chromosomes, normal centromeres, small chromosome number, uninucleated cells, diploid or haploid cells, sexual reproduction, long intermitotic period and slow rates of meiosis — are associated with high radiosensitivity (Sparrow 1962). Woody plants are about twice as sensitive as herbacious species (Sparrow & Sparrow 1965). Trees tend to be more sensitive than shrubs, which in turn are more sensitive than herbacious species such as grasses and forbs. Primitive forms, such as lichens, mosses and liverworts, are more resistant than vascular plants, while microflora can be even more so. Plants of low stature dominate communities exposed to harsh soil conditions or climatically extreme environments. Such plants have molecular and cellular characteristics that enhance their ability to tolerate stress, including that from ionizing radiation. A specific case is polyploidy, a condition common to species that survive extreme environments (Whicker & Fraley 1974), and one that also confers radioresistance (Sparrow 1962).

Apart from inherent radiosensitivity, it is important to consider the degree of protection afforded to meristematic tissues, the regions of active cell division at the growing tips of roots and shoots, and the flower bud. Species with exposed meristems or buds may receive much higher doses to these critical tissues than plants with growth or reproductive tissues that are underground or protected by thick scales.

Effects on animal populations

The impacts of radionuclides on animal populations are difficult to study, due to their mobility, secretive habits and dependence on the plant community. Early work focused on mortality of laboratory animals (mainly mammals and insects) following acute doses of X-rays or gamma rays (IAEA 1992). In the 1960s and 1970s, mammals and reptiles were chronically irradiated in their natural habitats (Turner 1975). This work showed that although acute doses in the range of 3–11 Gy and chronic doses greater than 0.1 Gy/day could cause significant mortality in mammals, somewhat lower doses could impair reproduction. For example, acute doses of only 0.2 Gy have lowered reproduction in female mice (Gowen & Stadler 1964) and chronic dose rates approaching 10 mGy/day might impact on reproduction in some mammals and reptiles (IAEA 1992). In an experiment in which lizards were maintained in a large enclosure in their natural habitat and chronically exposed to gamma rays at about 20 mGy/day, Turner et al (1971) showed that although initially no adverse effects were observed, the females of one species eventually became sterile and the population drifted toward extinction.

In aquatic ecosystems fish generally appear to be the most radiosensitive organisms, and gametogenesis and embryo development appear to be the most sensitive stages of the life cycle (IAEA 1976). In general, aquatic organisms tend to be comparable to their terrestrial counterparts in terms of radiosensitivity, although being poikilothermic, the expression time of radiation damage is temperature dependent. Reviews have concluded that chronic doses rates of less than 10 mGy/day to aquatic organisms are not likely to produce measurable impacts on populations (IAEA 1976, 1992).

The response of animal populations to radiation can be modified by stress, physiological condition and exposure to other contaminants. For example, the pika (*Ochotona princeps*), a small rodent that lives in mountain areas, was less likely to survive acute exposures when subject to the rigours of their natural habitat and competition from non-irradiated neighbouring pikas (Markham & Whicker 1970, 1971). Pikas are highly territorial, and this creates considerable stress. Another example is provided by Angelovic et al (1969), who showed that an estuarine fish could tolerate more radiation at the upper end of its temperature range at low salinity. An explanation of this result involved the effect of radiation in altering the osmoregulatory mechanism.

Contamination from the Chernobyl accident caused disruptions in nearby animal populations. The species diversity of litter microarthropods was reduced throughout 1987 in some forest areas within the 30 km zone, and juvenile invertebrates in areas receiving doses greater than 30 Gy were depleted (Krivolutsky & Pokarzhevsky 1990). Radionuclides tend to accumulate over time in the litter and near-surface soil, thus increasing the dose to animals living there. Mice populations in the more contaminated areas exhibited increased mortality, decreased reproduction and a variety of physiological disorders (Kryshev 1992). The numbers of mice reported in Kryshev's review ranged between 2–37% of normal, and fluctuated over a four-year period, suggesting population instability. Shevchenko et al (1992) found genetic disorders in mice that increased with dose. Radiogenic dominant lethal mutations in sperm stem cells led to embryonic mortality and sterility in males, causing a low frequency of subsequent genetic disorders. Reciprocal translocations in spermatocytes increased with dose, but their frequency was less than 1% in all dose groups. When exposed as embryos, however, the frequency was higher. Similar findings after the Kyshtym accident have been reported in animals (Krivolutsky et al 1993, Ilyenko & Krapivko 1993, Dubinin & Shevchenko 1976, Tikhomirov & Shcheglov 1994).

Recovery of radiation-damaged ecosystems

Biological communities damaged by radiation will recover, once the intensity of the dose rate becomes sufficiently reduced, provided that healthy propagules are available and that soil quality is adequate (Whicker & Fraley 1974). Obviously, the degree of damage affects recovery rate, as does size and shape of the damaged area. The smaller the area, the more rapid is seed and animal dispersal from unaffected areas. If the damaged area were large enough to delay vegetative succession seriously, soil would be lost through erosion and nutrient leaching would reduce fertility. Recovery of radiation-damaged ecosystems is similar to that from fire (Whicker & Fraley 1974).

Experience from the Kyshtym and Chernobyl accidents indicates that the most heavily impacted zones are showing substantial recovery. Based on work at Chernobyl, Arkhipov et al (1994), stated, 'Five years after the accident, forest stands inside the 10 km zone appeared to have restored their viability completely'. Production of herbacious plant seeds and their viability appeared relatively normal in the first three years after the accident at Chernobyl, suggesting that plant regeneration was possible (Taskaev et al 1992). Some 2.5 years after the accident, populations of soil fauna were recovering significantly and within three years, rodent populations were increasing, apparently due to immigration of animals from less-contaminated areas (Kryshev 1992). Evacuation of people from the 30 km exclusion zone around Chernobyl, and succession of abandoned agricultural fields toward natural meadow and forest, have led to increases in wild mammals and birds, and the general appearance of the area is now that of a nature preserve (Kryshev 1992). I have found no evidence in the literature of cases where a plant or animal species has been permanently eliminated from a radioactively contaminated natural ecosystem. On the other hand, there are examples where clean-up activities involving soil removal have altered ecosystems, perhaps permanently.

Areas that require research

Although many data have accumulated on the effects of large radionuclide releases on plants and animals, questions still remain. Most practical experience has centred on the coniferous forests and agricultural lands impacted by the Kyshtym and Chernobyl accidents. Many other ecosystems — such as arctic and alpine tundra, deserts and shrublands, and most freshwater and marine environments — have received little research. Almost no research on the radiosensitivity of aquatic macrophytes has been done. One might expect that the dosimetry involved in radionuclide contamination of the environment would be routine by now. However, this is not the case because each situation poses somewhat unique radionuclide distribution dynamics and morphology of critical tissues. The dosimetry of environmental radioactivity, particularly alpha and beta emissions, is far more complex than that of point gamma sources. Most large releases of radionuclides can be accompanied by other contaminants. Our knowledge of possible interacting effects of radiation and other physical and chemical stresses is weak.

I question whether we can be certain about the most sensitive, critical biological damage endpoints to quantify. Is reproduction, as indicated in the study by IAEA (1992), the most ecologically relevant endpoint? Is it possible that doses too low to affect reproduction might cause a sufficient mutation load in populations to alter their evolutionary course? Can we rely on molecular repair, lethal mutations and natural selection to restore the genetic integrity of radiation-impacted ecosystems? Present research might eventually answer some of these questions at Kyshtym and Chernobyl. This work should be continued for perhaps two decades longer to answer questions about recovery of genetic integrity. Experimental long-term work on other biological systems, using new methods of molecular biology combined with classical ecological measurements, should be carried out if our predictive power is to improve significantly.

Acknowledgements

This work was made possible by the Colorado State University and the Savannah River Ecology Laboratory through the Education, Research and Development Association of Georgia Universities and the Westinghouse Savannah River Company. The assistance of Randy Whicker in providing relevant literature is gratefully acknowledged.

References

Alexakhin RM 1993 Radioecological lessons of Chernobyl. Radiat Biol Ecol 33:73–80

Alexakhin RM, Karaban RT, Prister BS et al 1994 The effects of acute irradiation on a forest biogeocenosis: experimental data, model and practical applications for accidental cases. Sci Tot Environ 157:357–369

Angelovic JW, White JC, Davis EM 1969 Interactions of ionizing radiation, salinity, and temperature on the estuarine fish, *Fundulus heteroclitus*. In: Nelson DJ, Evans FC (eds) Symposium on radioecology. National Technical Information Service, Springfield, VA, p 131–141

Arkhipov NP, Kuchma ND, Askbrant S, Pasternak PS, Musica VV 1994 Acute and long-term effects of irradiation on pine (*Pinus silvestris*) stands post-Chernobyl. Sci Tot Environ 157:383–386

Barnthouse LW 1995 Effects of ionizing radiation on terrestrial plants and animals: a workshop report. National Technical Information Service, Springfield, VA, p 7–9

Dubinin NP, Shevchenko VA 1976 Mutation processes in irradiated natural populations. In: Mechanisms of genetic processes: mutagenesis and repair. Nauka, Moscow, p 265–291

Fraley L, Whicker FW 1973 Response of shortgrass plains vegetation to gamma radiation. Radiat Botany 13:331–353

Gowen JW, Stadler J 1964 Acute irradiation effects on reproductivity of different strains of mice. In: Carlson WD, Gassner FX (eds) Effects of ionizing radiation on the reproductive system. Pergamon, Oxford, p 45–58

IAEA 1976 Effects of ionizing radiation on aquatic organisms and ecosystems. International Atomic Energy Agency, Vienna (Technical Report Series 172)

IAEA 1992 Effects of ionizing radiation on plants and animals at levels implied by current radiation protection standards. International Atomic Energy Agency, Vienna (Technical Report Series 332)

Ilyenko AI, Krapivko TP 1993 Ecological consequences of radioactive contamination for populations of small mammals. In: Sokolov VE, Krivolutsky DA (eds) Ecological consequences of radioactive contamination in the southern Urals. Nauka, Moscow, p 171–180

Krivolutsky DA, Pokarzhevsky AD 1990 Changes in the population of soil fauna caused by the Chernobyl nuclear power plant accident. In: Biological and radioecological consequences of the accident at the Chernobyl nuclear power plant. Proceedings of the first international conference. Nauka, Moscow, p 78

Krivolutsky DA, Usachev BL, Arkhireyera AI et al 1993 Changes in the structure of animal populations (above-ground and soil invertebrates) as affected by contamination of land with strontium-90. In: Sokolov VE, Krivolutsky DA (eds) Ecological consequences of radioactive contamination in the southern Urals. Nauka, Moscow, p 241–249

Kryshev II 1992 Radioecological consequences of the Chernobyl accident. Nuclear Society International, Moscow

Léonard A, Delpoux M, Meyer R, Decat G, Léonard ED 1985 Effect of an enhanced natural radioactivity on mammal fertility. Sci Tot Environ 45:535–542

Markham OD, Whicker FW 1970 Radiation LD50$_{(30)}$ of pikas (*Ochotona princeps*) in the natural environment and in captivity. Am Midl Nat 84:248–252

Markham OD, Whicker FW 1971 Intraspecific competition and response of pikas (*Ochotona princeps*) to radiation. In: Nelson DJ (ed) Radionuclides in ecosystems, vol 2. National Technical Information Service, Springfield, VA, p 1070–1075

McClellan GE, Anno GH, Whicker FW 1994 Chernobyl doses, vol 1: Analysis of forest canopy radiation response from multispectral imagery and the relationship to doses. Defense Nuclear Agency, Alexandria, VA

Platt RB 1965 Ionizing radiation and homeostasis of ecosystems. In: Woodwell GM (ed) Ecological effects of nuclear war. Brookhaven National Laboratory, Upton, NY, p 39–60

Shevchenko VA, Pomerantseva MD, Ramaiya LK, Chekhovich AV, Testov BV 1992 Genetic disorders in mice exposed to radiation in the vicinity of the Chernobyl nuclear power station. Sci Tot Environ 112:45–56

Sparrow AH 1962 The role of the cell nucleus in determining radiosensitivity. Brookhaven National Laboratory, Upton, NY

Sparrow RC, Sparrow AH 1965 Relative radiosensitivities of woody and herbacious spermatophytes. Science 147:1449–1451

Sparrow AH, Woodwell GM 1963 Prediction of the sensitivity of plants to chronic gamma radiation. In: Schultz V, Klement AW Jr (eds) Radioecology. Reinhold, New York, p 257–270

Taskaev AI, Frolova NP, Popova ON, Shevchenko VA 1992 The monitoring of herbaceous seeds in the 30- km zone of the Chernobyl nuclear accident. Sci Tot Environ 112:57–67

Tikhomirov FA, Romanov GN 1993 Doses of radiation to organisms under conditions of radioactive contamination of a forest. In: Sokolov VE, Krivolutsky DA (eds) Ecological consequences of radioactive contamination in the southern Urals. Nauka, Moscow, p 13–20

Tikhomirov FA, Shcheglov AI 1994 Main investigation results on the forest radioecology in the Kyshtym and Chernobyl accident zones. Sci Tot Environ 157:45–57

Turner FB 1975 Effects of continuous irradiation on animal populations. Adv Radiat Biol 5:83–144

Turner FB, Licht P, Thrasher JD, Medica PA, Lannom JR 1971 Radiation-induced sterility in natural populations of lizards (*Crotaphytus wislizenii* and *Cnemidophorus tigris*). In: Nelson DJ (ed) Radionuclides in ecosystems, vol 2. National Technical Information Service, Springfield, VA, p 1131–1143

Whicker FW, Fraley L 1974 Effects of ionizing radiation on terrestrial plant communities. Adv Radiat Biol 4:317–366

Whicker FW, Schultz V 1982 Radioecology: nuclear energy and the environment. CRC Press, Boca Raton, FL

Woodwell GM 1967 Radiation and the patterns of nature. Science 156:461–470

DISCUSSION

Bauchinger: You mentioned that the recoveries after fire and radiation accidents are similar. However, this statement referred to short-term observations, so is it likely that it will also be true in the long-term?

Whicker: I'm not certain sure that anyone has followed it over a longer time period, so it is possible that there are some subtle differences. I was referring to gross apparent similarities, but there could be some subtle differences also in the short-term. If an area of 1 km^2 was denuded by radiation, certain plants would initially colonize the area, and others would later invade these colonizers. In time, these would die off and be succeeded by other plants. Ultimately, given enough time, the ecosystem would evolve back to what it originally was, and if the soil quality and climate were the same, there would also be a similar total productivity in terms of biomass. This process may take decades, or even longer.

Streffer: There are acute, immediate effects in the region exposed to the release of radionuclides, but in terms of a long-term effect, the migration of animal populations is more important

Whicker: Migration can complicate the interpretation, particularly in the case of chronic irradiation. Chronic irradiation of a community may cause reproductive changes and perhaps even mortality. On the other hand, if the area is relatively small and is surrounded by an unaffected area, then there is a natural tendency for unaffected individuals to move in and compete with affected individuals within the area.

Bauchinger: What cell types in the plants have been subjected to chromosomal analysis?

Whicker: Many cell types have been analysed, including the germ cells and cells from the meristems.

Frissel: Is it possible that adaptation to radiation stress may induce radiation resistance in the population for some period afterwards?

Whicker: I've come across that idea, but I don't fully understand the mechanism by which it could occur. If it were true, it would imply that the animals might have evolved enhanced repair mechanisms for genetic material that was susceptible to breaking. This idea sounds rather far-fetched to me, unless the animal population was mildly exposed for a long period of time.

Balonov: There have been some studies of mice radioresistance in the Kyshtym areas (see Ilyenko & Krapivko 1993). A couple of decades after the accident the radioresistance in mice was measured, and found to be at a higher level than in normal populations. However, the mechanism of genetic selection is not clear. Could you comment on this?

Whicker: I wish I could. I've read these papers and I don't know how to interpret the results.

Goldman: It is possible that the strains of mice present at the time of the accident vary in the degree of their radiosensitivity. Therefore, the genotype of the repopulated mouse strain may not be identical to what it was originally if radiation eliminated sensitive subpopulations from the breeding pool.

Whicker: But that's merely speculation. They did not show that the different strains were differentially radiosensitive.

Streffer: No one has shown that irradiation increases long-term radioresistance. There's no doubt that mouse strains have a high degree of variability in radioresistance, and clinical data have demonstrated that this is also the case for humans. It is possible that some selection occurs, but it is unlikely that radioresistance can increase over the long-term. Increased radioresistance in the short-term, however, has been shown in many systems. For example, in the haematopoietic system irradiation causes more blood cells to be produced in the short-term, which has the effect of increasing radioresistance. However, this increase in production and radioresistance decreases back to normal within a few weeks. In addition, many groups over the last few years have shown that a low dose of irradiation can cause an increased radioresistance of cells, so that if they are irradiated subsequently, they have fewer chromosomal aberrations than cells that were not given a prior dose (Wojcik & Streffer 1994). Again, this is only a short-term effect because the second irradiation has to be carried out within a few hours of the first.

Whicker: Are DNA repair enzymes involved in this?

Streffer: It has always been thought that DNA repair is induced, but no one has actually demonstrated this in mammalian cells. Also, the intra-individual variability in radioresistance is high. Therefore, there are many variables which we do not understand.

Goldman: Wolff et al (1988) showed that a small priming radiation dose given to T lymphocytes results in those T lymphocytes having a much more radiation-resistant survival curve than those cells that didn't first receive the priming dose. Again, it is not a long-lasting phenomenon.

There are also several reports of certain crops which, following low dose radiation exposures, outproduce the crops that have not been exposed. This is sometimes referred to as hormesis, a beneficial effect of low doses of agents that produce adverse effects at high doses (Luckey 1980).

Roed: In order to cause damage to DNA, chemical agents have to cross many barriers, but this is not the case for physical agents. I do not understand how the DNA could be physically protected by prior irradiation.

Streffer: We irradiate the cell with physical agents that cause chromosome breaks. The chromosomal damage is repaired quickly, i.e. within minutes. When we observe the chromosome aberrations some hours later, only 1–5% of the damage remains. It is possible that radioresistance is achieved by making this repair more efficient so that only 0.5% of the damage remains. In most mammalian cells the DNA repair system is already optimally efficient, so that it is impossible to increase efficiency under those conditions. However, gene expression is induced by small radiation doses, so new enzymes may be formed that are somehow involved in increasing radioresistance by repairing damage more efficiently.

Paretzke: How can you explain the observation that irradiated mice have an increased survival time along those lines?

Streffer: It is possible that the haemopoietic system becomes more active as a result of low dose irradiation, so that there is a higher proportion of stem cells that produce blood cells more rapidly. The haemopoietic system is the most critical system with respect to radiation sickness, so if it becomes more efficient at renewing blood cells then the mouse could become more radioresistant. This effect has been demonstrated, but it is only a short-term effect (Dacquisto & Major 1959). Irradiation may also cause changes to the immunological system, but nothing is known at present how this could increase radioresistance.

Whicker: These mice received doses of 1–8 Gy, and they exhibited many symptoms of radiation sickness. Only a fraction of them survived this dose. However, the extra energy requirement for escaping predators or for competing with other animals for space was possibly sufficient to cause additional mortality.

Goldman: There have been many studies on radiation dose priming in rodents. Many studies have suggested that there's no difference in cancer incidence and life expectancy versus the unexposed animals at low dose rates, and that it increases at intermediate and high dose rates. There was an erroneous idea, based on the early work of E. Lorenz during the second world war, that rodents exposed to low dose irradiation lived longer and had fewer cancers than in the control group (Lorenz 1950). However, when this work was reviewed carefully, it was discovered that the control mice were kept in a different environment which had a different temperature. When the experiment was repeated with all the rodents kept at the same temperature, there were no differences between the experimental and control group.

Bauchinger: You mentioned that there was a relationship between radiation sensitivity and the chromosome size. Were you referring to chromosome size in terms of metaphase length or to DNA content? I'm asking this because there is some contrary evidence for human lymphocytes irradiated *in vitro* with 3 Gy X-rays, i.e. that larger chromosomes tend to be less involved in translocations than would be expected from their DNA content, and those with a lower DNA content showed a relatively higher involvement (Knehr et al 1994).

Whicker: I don't know the answer to that. The way I've always thought about it, as a layman in this subject, is that if I was going to organize all of my genetic information, would I want to have it in a few large strands of DNA or in many smaller strands? If the same dose is given in both cases, one would expect the same number of breaks, but if a break occurs in a large strand, then there is a greater chance of losing more information than if a smaller strand is broken.

Goldman: Sparrow et al (1967) made a plot of individual plant chromosome volume against median lethal dose and the relationship was a straight line over seven orders of magnitude. The plants with the largest chromosomes were the conifers, and the deciduous trees had smaller chromosomes. Conifers are the most sensitive, with their median lethal radiation dose of about 6 Gy, which is similar to humans.

Konoplev: Ecosystems in contaminated areas of the USA are rather different from those in Russia. Did you identify any specific differences that arose as a result of these differences in the ecosystem types?

Whicker: But there are many similarities between the study sites at Brookhaven National Laboratory, where there is an oak/pine forest, and Chernobyl, in terms of the general climate and types of plants that are present (Woodwell 1967). In fact, the area around the Savannah River site has pines, hardwoods and sandy soils, although the climate there is warmer.

Renn: Is there any animal that is able to sensor radioactive exposure and thus be prepared to flee from the area? This would be an interesting observation from an evolutionary point of view.

Whicker: I cannot speak knowledgeably on this, except that I do have one anecdotal report. There was an unpublished study at the Savannah River site many years ago in which bobcats were trapped and irradiated. The bobcats went berserk when the source was turned on. Apparently, the bobcat could somehow sense something, perhaps it could smell the ozone produced in the air. However, in the studies that I'm familiar with the animals have no apparent sensory perception of radiation.

References

Dacquisto MP, Major MC 1959 Acquired radioresistance. A review of the literature and report of a confirmatory experiment. Radiat Res 10:118–129

Ilyenko AI, Krapivko TP 1993 Ecological consequences of radioactive contamination for populations of small mammals. In: Sokolov VE, Krivolutsky DA (eds) Ecological consequences of radioactive contamination in the Southern Urals. Nauka, Moscow, p 171–180

Knehr S, Zitzelsberger H, Braselmann H, Bauchinger M 1994 Analysis for DNA-proportional distribution of radiation-induced chromosome aberrations in various triple combinations of human chromosomes using fluorescence *in situ* hybridization. Int J Radiat Biol 65:683–690

Luckey TD 1980 Radiation hormesis, CRC Press, Boca Raton, FL

Lorenz E 1950 Some biologic effects of long continued irradiation. Am J Roentgenol Radium Therapy Nucl Med 63:176–185

Sparrow AH, Underbrink AG, Sparrow RC 1967 Chromosomes and cellular radiosensitivity. I. Radiation research 32:915–945

Wojcik A, Streffer C 1994 Adaptive response to ionizing radiation in mammalian cells: a review. Biol Zentrabl 113:417–434

Woodwell GM 1967 Radiation and the patterns of nature. Science 156:461–470

Wolff S, Afzal V, Wiencke JK, Oliveri G, Michaeli A 1988 Human lymphocytes exposed to low doses of ionizing radiations become refractory to high doses of radiation as well as to chemical mutagens that induce double-strand breaks in DNA. Int J Rad Biol Rel Stud Phys Chem Med 53:39–47

General discussion II

Goldman: I have some infrared satellite images of the damage to the pine forest some 8–10 km west of the Chernobyl reactor, which were taken weekly by the Landsat 4 Thematic Mapper Satellite. By enhancing the infrared reflectance wavelengths for the bands corresponding to chlorophyll and moisture we have been able to discern living from dead trees, and from an altitude of about 500 km we have been able to develop a crude spatial and temporal map of the region that was hit the heaviest. Since pine trees have about a 6 Gy median lethal dose, the images, starting about three weeks after the accident, indicated a western swath of dying and dead trees, the so-called 'red forest'. I later learned that the map was correct but the doses were not. The trees had received doses of over 100 Gy, but regardless of the dose, the technique at least showed where the doses exceeded a 6 Gy detection threshold. Over the next 10 years, much of the damaged forest that was not cut down has shown major regrowth and repair. The more resistant deciduous trees showed much less radiation damage.

Frissel: What is a good criterion for an ecosystem? An ecosystem restores itself unless the primary production of the dominant vegetation is damaged. Would it be fair to say that the ecosystem is not seriously damaged as long as the primary production is not damaged?

Whicker: Yes, it would be fair to say that.

Håkanson: There are many ways of defining an ecosystem, which is a complex unit with many chemical, physical and biological components. A threat, such as the release or fallout of radiocaesium, can then be added to that complexity. We would like to measure or predict the effects of this fallout on the ecosystem, which are also extremely complicated. There are, however, some basic rules that one can apply. For example, the biological parts of the ecosystem can be regarded as an eco-chain, and the weakest part of the chain, i.e. the organisms that are most sensitive to the threat, can be identified. If those key functional organisms are eliminated, a completely different ecosystem develops. In my opinion, a good operational method is to study the most sensitive organisms, rather than all of them because this would take too long.

Whicker: A simple example of this is a natural ecosystem dominated by pines because they affect the other species present and they are also radiosensitive.

Paretzke: I would also like to mention that Ward Whicker is the chairman of a new report committee dealing with the statistical aspects of environmental sampling in the field of radioecology. How is 'a representative sample' chosen in practice? Which aspects must be considered and what are the limitations? We are hoping that they will issue a report answering these questions in a couple of years time.

Streffer: The reproduction of mammals is also a sensitive parameter. I would like to ask Ward Whicker where he obtained his figures of 0.3 Gy and 0.01 Gy/day for the levels of acute and chronic irradiation, respectively, that affect reproduction.

Whicker: These are, in part, from experimental data generated by Fred Turner and colleagues many years ago at the Nevada test site (Turner et al 1971). They had a large enclosure that contained two species of lizard and some small mammals. There was a fence around this enclosure so that these animals could not get out and other animals could not get in. They erected a tower and irradiated the animals using a point source which was shielded in such a way so that the irradiation dose rate over the whole area was roughly constant at about 0.02 Gy/day. They found that there was no impact on mortality. However, in one species of lizard the females ultimately became sterile, and after about six to seven years the lizards were drifting toward extinction.

There was also another study by French et al (1974) in which they chronically irradiated wild desert rodents in the laboratory. I believe that they were able to show impaired reproduction at dose rates approaching values as low as 10 mGy/day.

Cigna: One of the basic principles of radiation protection is the compliance with the individual limits, i.e. not a single person should be exposed to a dose higher than the limit itself. Within an ecosystem, the preservation of the population of each species of organisms must be assured and not the preservation of each single individual. For example, the destruction of some organisms is normally accepted when clearing parts of a forest for agricultural or construction purposes. Therefore, there are no reasons to treat the effects of ionizing radiation differently than the effects of any other human action. For this reason, the protection of the environment is generally assured when the criteria of radiation protection, established for humans, are applied. There could be some theoretical exceptions to this rule when, for example, a discharge of radioactive effluents is planned in a totally uninhabited area. However, in practice, other constraints would avoid such an occurrence.

Paretzke: I would like to ask Asker Aarkrog what his opinion is of the underground testing being carried out at the Mururoa Atoll?

Aarkrog: Many of us have been asked about the consequences of these tests. The general belief among marine radioecologists is that they will not harm the marine environment, even if there is a release of radionuclides. Such a release would have less damaging effects than a release from a real underwater explosion, such as the one that occurred at Bikini Atoll, for example. I had a discussion some time ago with a Danish 'environmentalist', who claimed that underground explosions will have environmental consequences because the lithosere will be affected. This line of argument considers the total environment, including the abiotic environment, as being precious and therefore, if this point of view is accepted, underground explosions are unacceptable.

Howard: The International Commission on Radiological Protection initially suggested that if humans are protected from ionizing radiation, then the environment is also protected. What are the current views on this?

Paretzke: Five years ago an advisory group of the International Atomic Energy Agency met in Vienna to issue a report. They made an assessment of doses to plants and to terrestrial and aquatic animals from radionuclides in the environment. For most radionuclides, protecting humans via all possible pathways with an annual dose limit of 1 mSv resulted in a protective effect for all the animals. One exception to this, however, might be plutonium, which does not enter the human food-chain easily and can be directly ingested by some animals. Strontium may also be an exception.

Whicker: Populations that may not be adequately protected may include endangered species and species with long life spans which take a long time to reach reproductive age. Such populations may be sensitive to chronic radiation, and a few individuals could be important for the perpetuation of the species. We have to be more careful about situations such as these.

Balonov: The question of protecting humans and the environment is different for large releases of radionuclides, such as at Chernobyl, because most humans are evacuated from contaminated areas. In these areas there are major effects on the environment, so if we want to protect these environments, perhaps we should consider special countermeasures to protect the animals. For example, perhaps some sort of generator could be switched on so that the animals run away from the area.

Whicker: In our study we didn't take accidents into account because we were more concerned about the laws to prevent routine nuclear releases from having harmful effects on humans and their environments. I imagine that it's not possible or realistic to set up laws to protect against accidents or acts of aggression.

Frissel: I have some doubts as to whether the assumption that the environment is protected if humans are protected is correct. There may be ecosystems that we have not considered. For example, in Botswana lions feed almost entirely on buffalos. I have seen these buffalos grazing and I was surprised to see how much particulate soil matter they consume. If these areas were contaminated, they would accumulate large amounts of radioactivity. Humans are absent or almost absent in such areas, so an assessment calculation is meaningless. Moreover, the accepted idea is that we have to protect individual humans, but for animals we only have to protect the animal population as a whole, i.e. individual losses of animals are not important. This might be true for most animals, but certainly not for rare species or small animal populations.

Whicker: We made a couple of assumptions in our study. We assumed that we were dealing only with environments in which humans inhabit and derive their sustenance, so that if there was a contamination event, we could calculate the doses received by humans. Protecting humans by 1 mSv per year also assumes a certain amount of deposition. We then asked what is the dose received by plants and animals by that certain amount of deposition, and we found that it was two to three orders of magnitude below the dose which is known to affect reproduction in the most sensitive plants and animals that have been studied. The strongest reason for this apparent discrepancy involves our yardstick for measuring effects. That is, we have a conservative attitude towards protecting the individual person; however, when we're dealing with the natural environment, we worry about the population and not the individual.

I would also like to tell you about a situation that's happening in the USA. I don't know how many of you are also facing a similar problem. In the USA there has been a large push to clean up contaminated ecosystems that have resulted from the cold war. The Savannah River site, Hanford, Los Almos, Rocky Flats and Oak Ridge are some of the areas that have low levels of contamination. These environments have been protected from human habitation for 40 years, and they have become valuable wildlife sanctuaries. There has been talk of spending over $US500 billion over the next 30 years to clean up these areas, but a bulldozer will do far more damage to the ecosystem than low-level irradiation and it will cost the taxpayers billions of dollars. Some politicians want to do this because it sounds good. They stand more of a chance of being elected if they bring money into these communities for the clean-up operations. We would first like to see rigorous risk analyses being done on these ecosystems, so that we can determine whether they really need to be cleaned up. We need to determine whether these ecological effects are significant, and we need to demonstrate that if the landuse changes in the future, for instance if a farmer decides to live and work there, that the risks will be acceptable.

Let me tell you another story about the Savannah River site. If one canoes down the Savannah River, on one side one would see five nuclear reactors and two fuel separation and reprocessing facilities. These all have small effluents that empty into tributaries of the Savannah River, and the public worries about these streams and the impact of radionuclides. However, they are some of the only streams that empty into the river which are essentially clean — they contain lots of organic matter and virtually no pollutants, except a very small amount of caesium, strontium and tritium. On the other side of the river there are numerous streams that contain agricultural run-off, which has high levels of pesticides, fertilizer and silt. Yet, people are more worried about the radioactivity.

Gadd: I can empathize with lay people thinking that mud is less dangerous than radionuclides. There are a number of possible reasons for this: the radioecologists may not be educating the public adequately, but more likely, the public will not believe them anyway.

Whicker: I speak to public groups all the time, and there's a certain group of people that only believe what they want to believe and they will try to destroy your credibility no matter what you say, unless you say that plutonium causes cancer so that they can obtain some money through litigation. You can't go into most public meetings and expect to be treated as a credible witness, no matter who you are or what you say. You have to earn credibility by spending a lot of time and effort with the public, such as inviting them to your laboratory and showing them that you're a human being too. It is quite possible to educate the people who care about the truth and to change their minds.

Roed: It has been shown that all the large releases of radionuclides have not seriously damaged the environment, but problems may occur if we damage the environment in order to protect ourselves from small amounts of radiation, i.e. the decontamination of the environment can be more damaging than the irradiation itself.

Whicker: I have another example of this. Most of the plutonium deposits at Rocky Flats in Colorado were due to remediation. When the leaking oil drums were cleaned up, the contaminated soil was moved around by high winds. This mistake has been made three or four times, and each time more plutonium is released. The public is not aware of this, and many people still think that the clean-up operation was a good thing.

Goldman: This concerns a fundamental issue, which is that most people believe that every radiation dose has a proportional radiation risk, and that there's no such a thing as a dose so small that there's no risk. Secondly, when it comes to the practicality of cleaning up, we don't know to what level this can be done because of the drive to revert to nature. Perhaps a clean-up should be done when there could be adverse consequences that can be averted. One cannot prove that there's going to be any improvement in the public health potential for the future for any part of the ecosystem. There may be a practical contamination threshold decision point. The cost of completely restoring an entire contaminated region is too high for such an option to be viable, even for the areas in the USA that are most heavily contaminated. It won't happen.

Aarkrog: I would like to give another example of restoring the environment. At Thule in northwest Greenland, where a B-52 crashed on the sea ice in 1968, 0.5 kg plutonium was deposited on the bottom of the sea at a depth of about 200 m and covering an area of about 100 km². The people in Greenland want this area to be cleaned up by the USA. It seems unlikely that 0.5 kg plutonium on the bottom of the sea would be of any harm to this arctic environment. From expeditions to Thule we know that the plutonium is buried by sediments deposited from melting icebergs. Furthermore, the biota from the seabed is not eaten directly by the local population. A clean-up operation would thus do more harm than good to this environment, and it would also be excessively costly.

Streffer: Many unreasonable things happen in the field of radioecology and its interpretation. However, we have to be careful that we are not misunderstood if we say that the Chernobyl accident did not harm the environment. There was certainly much damage to the environment around the nuclear power plant. Some people have died as a result of receiving acute radiation, and there have also been a number of effects on human health. We have to make it quite clear that we do not want this accident to be repeated, and we should do everything we can to minimize the release of radionuclides into the environment.

References

French NR, Maza BG, Hill HO, Aschwanden AP, Kaaz HW 1974 A population study of irradiated desert rodents. Ecol Monogr 44:45–68

Turner FB, Licht P, Thrasher JD, Medica PA, Lannom JR 1971 Radiation-induced sterility in natural populations of lizards (*Crotaphytus wislizenii* and *Cnemidophorus tigris*). In: Nelson DJ (ed) Radionuclides in ecosystems, vol 2. National Technical Information Service, Springfield, VA, p 1131–1143

Roles of micro-organisms in the environmental fate of radionuclides

G. M. Gadd

Department of Biological Sciences, University of Dundee, Dundee, DD1 4HN, UK

Abstract. Micro-organisms play important roles in the environmental fate of radionuclides in both aquatic and terrestrial ecosystems, with a multiplicity of physico-chemical and biological mechanisms effecting changes in mobility and speciation. Physico-chemical mechanisms of removal, which may be encompassed by the general term 'biosorption', include adsorption, ion exchange and entrapment. These are features of living and dead organisms as well as their derived products. In living cells biosorptive processes can be directly and indirectly influenced by metabolism, and may be reversible and affected by changing environmental conditions. Metabolism-dependent mechanisms of radionuclide immobilization include metal precipitation as sulfides, sequestration by metal-binding proteins and peptides, and transport and intracellular compartmentation. Chemical transformations of radionuclide species, particularly by reduction, can result in immobilization. Microbial processes involved in solubilization include autotrophic and heterotrophic leaching, complexation by siderophores and other metabolites, and chemical transformations. Such mechanisms are important components of natural biogeochemical cycles for radionuclides and should be considered in any analyses of environmental radionuclide contamination. Several micro-organism-based biotechnologies, e.g. those based on biosorption or precipitation, are of potential use for the treatment of radionuclide contamination.

1997 Health impacts of large releases of radionuclides. Wiley, Chichester (Ciba Foundation Symposium 203) p 94–108

Pollution of the environment by radionuclides arises as a result of many activities, which are largely industrial. These pollutants are discharged or transported into the atmosphere, and aquatic and terrestrial environments, and may reach high concentrations, especially near the site of entry. Metallic radionuclides have also entered the environment as a result of weapons testing and accidents such as Chernobyl. The fate and effects of radionuclides in ecosystems is not well understood but concerns over transfer along aquatic and terrestrial food-chains are of economic and public health significance. Elevated environmental awareness among consumers and industrialists, and increasingly strict legal constraints on emissions, have led to an increased need for cost-effective emission control as well as additional methods for treatment of contaminated materials (Macaskie & Dean 1989, Brierley 1990, Volesky 1990, Gadd 1988, 1992, White et al 1995).

Once in the environment, radionuclides may undergo numerous transformations into a variety of mobile and immobile forms (Fig. 1). While abiotic environmental parameters are of great significance in determining the environmental fate of radionuclides, microbiological activity is also important and can account for a large number of the environmental fates of radionuclides as well as affecting radionuclide interactions with organic and inorganic components of the environment. Micro-organisms are at the beginning (primary producers) and end (consumers, decomposers) of almost all food-chains, and they play major roles in virtually all biogeochemical cycles. Radionuclides can be bound or precipitated by microbial products and metabolites, or accumulated by cells by non-specific physico-chemical interactions, specific mechanisms of sequestration or transport. A variety of oxidation–reduction reactions also affect radionuclide speciation and mobility (Beveridge & Doyle 1989, Gadd 1988, 1992, 1993a,b, Lovley 1993, 1995, White et al 1995). This chapter highlights the roles played by micro-organisms in the environmental fate of metallic radionuclides. Fundamental mechanisms underlying radionuclide immobilization, transformation or solubilization are outlined with a brief discussion of their biotechnological potential for treatment of contaminated wastes. The author has published several other detailed accounts of this topic (Gadd 1988, 1992, 1993a,b, Avery et al 1992, Gadd & White 1993, Tobin et al 1994, White et al 1995).

Microbial processes involved in the environmental fate of radionuclides

Biotransformations of metallic radionuclides by micro-organisms are of great importance in the biosphere and have additional applications for bioremediation (Gadd 1992, 1993b, Gadd & White 1993, White et al 1995). Reactions that are mediated by micro-organisms include the solubilization of metals from minerals by the production of acids or chelating agents (Francis 1990, 1994, Francis et al 1992, Morley et al 1996), and the removal of metals from aqueous solution. A number of mechanisms are involved in this removal including biosorption, accumulation and chemical precipitation, e.g. as sulfides. Chemical transformations such as oxidation, reduction, alkylation or dealkylation are also catalysed by a wide range of micro-organisms. These reactions greatly alter a number of important parameters—such as toxicity, volatility and water solubility—that influence biotic effects and environmental mobility (Fig. 1) (Gadd 1992, 1993b).

Radionuclide immobilization by micro-organisms

Biosorption and accumulation

Biosorption can be defined as radionuclide uptake by micro-organisms by physico-chemical mechanisms, such as adsorption or ion exchange. However, in living cells metabolic activity may also influence and/or contribute to the process. Biosorption

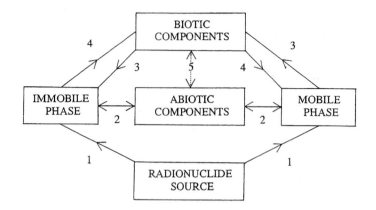

FIG. 1. Diagrammatic model depicting the roles of micro-organisms in the environmental fate of radionuclides. The scheme is not exhaustive, but the major influence of micro-organisms in effecting transformations between soluble and insoluble phases is emphasized. The relative balance between such processes will depend on the environment and associated physico-chemical conditions and the micro-organism(s) involved, as well as relationships with plants, animals and anthropogenic activities. (1) Radionuclide deposition or entry into aerial, aquatic and terrestrial ecosystems as a result of, e.g. industrial activity, accidents, discharges, medical and chemical wastes, weapons testing and natural biogeochemical cycles. (2) Chemical equilibria between soluble and insoluble phases is influenced by abiotic components, including dead biota and their decomposition products, as well as other physico-chemical components of the environmental matrix, e.g. pH, water, inorganic and organic ions, molecules, compounds, colloids and particulates. (3) Immobilization by: biosorption to cell walls, exopolymers, other structural components and derived/excreted products; precipitation as a result of sulfide formation or reduction; other oxidative–reductive transformations; transport, accumulation, intracellular deposition, localization and sequestration; and adsorption and entrapment of colloids and particulates. (4) Mobilization of radionuclides by: autotrophic leaching; heterotrophic leaching; metabolite excretion including H^+ and organic acids; siderophores and other complexing agents; oxidative–reductive reactions; alkylation; and biodegradation of organo-radionuclide complexes. (5) Reciprocal interactions between biotic and abiotic components of the ecosystem. Includes: the balance between life, death and excretion; abiotic influence on microbial diversity, numbers and metabolic activity; the ingestion of particulates and colloids (including bacteria) by phagotrophic microbial eukaryotes (mainly protozoa); and the biotic modification of physico-chemical parameters including redox potential, pH, O_2, CO_2, other gases and metabolites, temperature, and nutrient depletion.

can also provide nucleation and stimulate the formation of extremely stable minerals (Beveridge & Doyle 1989). Almost all biological macromolecules have some affinity for radionuclides, with constituents of microbial cell walls and associated materials being of the greatest significance in biosorption. In addition, cationic forms of radionuclides, especially those of essential metals or essential metal 'mimics', can be transported into cells by transport systems of varying specificity. Once inside cells, metal radionuclides may be bound, precipitated or localized within intracellular structures or organelles, depending on the element concerned and the organism.

Biosorption by cell walls and associated components.   Microbial exopolymers that have received most attention in relation to metal and radionuclide binding are those which form capsules or slime layers. Most of these are composed of polysaccharides, glycoproteins and lipopolysaccharides, which may all be associated with protein. Bacterial cell walls have several components that contribute to general biosorptive processes. The carboxyl groups of the peptidoglycans are the main binding site in Gram-positive cell walls, with phosphate groups contributing significantly in Gram-negative organisms (Beveridge & Doyle 1989). Many fungi have a high chitin content in cell walls, and this polymer of N-acetyl glucosamine is an effective radionuclide biosorbent, as are chitosan and other chitin derivatives (Macaskie & Dean 1990, Tobin et al 1994). Actinide accumulation in intact fungal biomass appears mainly to comprise metabolism-independent biosorption to the cell wall (Gadd & White 1990, Volesky 1990, Tobin et al 1994). Fungal phenolic polymers and melanins possess many potential metal-binding sites. Oxygen-containing groups in these substances, including carboxyl, phenolic and alcoholic hydroxyl, carbonyl and methoxyl groups may be particularly important (Gadd 1993a).

Transport, accumulation and intracellular fate.   Many radionuclides, particularly cationic species of, for example, manganese, strontium, cobalt and zinc, can be transported into prokaryotic and eukaryotic micro-organisms. The consequences of radionuclide transport into microbial cells have been particularly explored in the case of radiocaesium. Micro-organisms from all major groups can accumulate caesium, and entry usually occurs via active transport systems for K^+ or sometimes other monovalent cations, e.g. NH_4^+ (Avery et al 1992). Caesium accumulation is dependent on factors such as external pH and monovalent cation concentration, especially K^+ (Avery et al 1992, Perkins & Gadd 1995). Caesium appears to be relatively non-toxic towards micro-organisms and accumulation may have an influence on environmental fate. Microbially associated caesium is believed to account for a significant proportion of total radioactive caesium in contaminated upland soils and forest organic layers (Dighton & Terry 1996). In addition, microbial decomposition of litter can result in mobilization of associated caesium (see Avery 1996). In the aquatic environment biotic processes also contribute to caesium cycling, and primary producers, i.e. cyanobacteria and algae, are capable of accumulating caesium (Avery et al 1992).

   In eukaryotic micro-organisms vacuoles appear to be a preferential intracellular location for caesium (Gadd 1993a, Avery 1995). This organelle is also the reservoir for certain other metals, e.g. cobalt, zinc, strontium and manganese (Gadd 1993a). Metals/radionuclides may also be precipitated within cells/organelles as sulfides, oxides and phosphates. Some intracellular biomolecules function specifically to bind toxic metals and are induced by their presence. Metal-binding proteins and peptides have been recorded in all microbial groups examined and it is conceivable that these may also have a role in the intracellular fate of metal radionuclides. Metallothioneins are small cysteine-rich polypeptides that can bind copper and zinc, for example, as well as non-essential metals like cadmium (Mehra & Winge 1991). Metal γ-glutamyl peptides (phytochelatins) are short peptides involved in metal detoxification in algae, plants, and some fungi and yeasts (Mehra & Winge 1991, Gadd 1993a).

Metal accumulation by macrofungi.   Elevated concentrations of radionuclides can occur in the fruiting bodies of higher fungi when growing in polluted environments, a phenomenon of social significance because of the widespread consumption of wild fungi in many countries. There have been several studies on the accumulation of radiocaesium (mainly ^{137}Cs) by macrofungi, particularly following the Chernobyl accident in 1986. Saprotrophic and mycorrhizal basidiomycetes can accumulate radiocaesium. These organisms may form a major pool of radiocaesium in the soil; grazing of fruit bodies by animals may lead to radiocaesium transfer along the food-chain (Dighton & Terry 1996). Deviations in the [137]Cs : [134]Cs ratio attributable to Chernobyl have revealed that there was considerable accumulation of pre-Chernobyl caesium probably from weapons testing. Radiocaesium accumulation in basidiomycetes appears species dependent, with influences exerted by soil properties. Radiocaesium influx rates into hyphae of several basidiomycetes showed considerable variation, with saprotrophic species exhibiting highest rates and mycorrhizal species the lowest (Dighton & Terry 1996).

Biodegradation of organo-radionuclide complexes.   Chelating agents are used for decontamination purposes and these can increase the solubility of radionuclides. Microbial degradation of radionuclide complexes may result in the release of the radionuclides and subsequent transformation into, for example, hydroxides, oxides or other compounds of lower solubility (Francis 1990, Francis et al 1992).

Reduction and precipitation

Apart from the biosorptive, accumulative and metabolic interactions described above, chemical reduction and/or precipitation of metals are the other main mechanisms of radionuclide immobilization leading to mineral and sulfide formation.

Reduction.   Reduction is one of the most important microbial biotransformations of metallic elements that can affect solubility. Dissimilatory reductive processes are carried out under anaerobic conditions and the micro-organisms involved are almost entirely obligate anaerobes. In this process, the oxidized form of the metal or metalloid element serves as the terminal electron acceptor for respiration. A strain of *Shewanella (Alteromonas) putrefaciens* that reduced Fe(III) and Mn(IV) also reduced U(VI) to U(IV) (Lovley et al 1991). Due to the low solubility of U(IV), the reaction was accompanied by the formation of a black precipitate of U(IV) carbonate. When the organisms were contained by dialysis tubing, the precipitate was associated with the organisms, indicating that it was the result of an enzymic reaction rather than reduction by reduced products (Lovley 1995). U(VI) was also reduced by the sulfate-reducing bacterium *Desulphovibrio desulphuricans* utilizing a mechanism that involved the electron transport chain, although the organism could not utilize U(VI) as an electron acceptor for growth (Lovley & Phillips 1992). Non-dissimilatory reductive processes are carried out by a wide range of organisms using metabolic reductant to reduce metal(loids); for example, as a component of an uptake process. However, this type of process may also occur in organisms adapted to environments having a high concentration of toxic metals, where it provides a mechanism of metal detoxification and resistance.

Sulfide precipitation.   Hydrogen sulfide is produced by sulfate-reducing bacteria, e.g. *Desulphovibrio* and *Desulphotomaculum* sp. The solubility products of most metal sulfides are extremely low and they are readily precipitated as sulfides, e.g. ZnS, CdS, CuS and FeS. Sulfate-reducing activity can occur as a result of anaerobic biomass decay and sulfidic immobilization of toxic metals, and radionuclides can occur in wastes and sediments as well as in biological treatment systems (Brierley 1990, White et al 1995, Fortin et al 1995) (see below).

Radionuclide solubilization by micro-organisms

A variety of microbial processes may increase radionuclide mobility. These are phenomena of particular significance in the terrestrial environment, with implications for transfer to plants and higher organisms as well as to the aquatic environment. Such processes may occur in contaminated sites as well as in wastes (Francis 1990), and they include autotrophic and heterotrophic leaching, the production of complexing agents and metabolites, and chemical transformations.

Autotrophic leaching

Much of the information on microbial leaching deals primarily with the oxidation of mineral ores by autotrophic bacteria under aerobic conditions. Such processes, catalysed chiefly by thiobacilli, e.g. *Thiobacillus ferrooxidans,* are used on a commercial scale for extraction of metals and uranium from ores, and metal recovery from wastes. It is likely that such a leaching process would also mobilize contaminating radionuclides in the soil. Iron- and sulfur-oxidizing bacteria are known to be important in solubilization of uranium from ores, mill tailings and coal wastes (Francis 1990).

Heterotrophic leaching

Heterotrophic bacteria and fungi can mediate radionuclide solubilization by several processes, including the production of protons, organic acids and chelating agents

(Morley et al 1996). Microbially produced dicarboxylic acids, gluconic acids, protocatechuic acid and salicylic acid are efficient chelators of metallic species and can accelerate metal mobility in soil. Soluble low molecular weight organo-uranyl complexes of UO_2^{2+} with organic acids including citric, oxalic, isocitric and succinic acids can be formed via carboxylic and phenolic groups (Francis 1990).

Siderophores

Siderophores are low molecular weight Fe(III) coordination compounds that are excreted under iron-limiting conditions by micro-organisms, particularly bacteria and fungi, to enable accumulation of iron from the environment. Although virtually specific for Fe(III), siderophores and analogous compounds can complex certain other metals, e.g. Ga(III), Cr(III), scandium, indium, nickel, uranium and thorium (Macaskie & Dean 1990). Plutonium can also be complexed by siderophores and a potential for actinide treatment has been suggested particularly as Pu(IV) and Fe(III) exhibit some similar chemical properties (Birch & Bachofen 1990).

Reduction

In contrast to the radionuclide immobilization described earlier, the solubility of certain other radionuclides may be increased by reduction, and this may favour their removal from matrices such as soils. For example, iron-reducing bacterial strains solubilized 40% of the plutonium present in contaminated soils within six to seven days (Rusin et al 1994). In a more extensive study, both iron- and sulfate-reducing bacteria were able to solubilize radium from uranium mine tailings, although the main mechanism appears to have been disruption of reducible host minerals (Landa & Gray 1995).

Microbial processes for treatment of radionuclide contamination

Most microbial systems explored to date are directed towards the treatment of liquid waste effluents or leachates (Macaskie & Dean 1989, Macaskie 1991, Gadd 1988, 1992), although there is increasing appreciation of *in situ* treatment methods, albeit mostly related to toxic metals, e.g. wetlands and stream meanders (see Gadd & White 1993).

Biosorption

Fungi and yeasts have received attention in connection with metal biosorption particularly because waste fungal biomass arises as a by-product from several industrial fermentations (Gadd 1990, Volesky 1990, Gadd & White 1990, Tobin et al 1994), whereas algae (including macroalgae) can be viewed as a renewable source of metal-sorbing biomass (Gadd 1988). Immobilized living biomass has mainly taken the form of biofilms on supports made of a range of inert materials. These have been used in a variety of bioreactor configurations, including rotating biological contactors, fixed bed reactors, trickle filters, fluidized beds and air-lift bioreactors (Gadd 1988, Macaskie & Dean 1989). As well as biofilms, living or dead biomass of all groups has been immobilized by encapsulation or cross-linking (Brierley et al 1989, Brierley 1990, de Rome & Gadd 1991, Tobin et al 1994). Supports include agar, cellulose, alginates, cross-linked ethyl acrylate–ethylene glycol dimethylacrylate, polyacrylamide, silica gel and the cross-linking reagents toluene diisocyanate and glutaraldehyde.

Precipitation

The main applications of microbially mediated precipitation of radionuclides are those involving sulfide precipitation, phosphatase-mediated precipitation and chemical reduction.

Sulfide precipitation. A purpose-designed, sludge-blanket reactor using sulfate-reducing bacteria has been developed by Shell Research Ltd and Budelco B.V. (Barnes et al 1992). This plant successfully removed toxic metals and sulfate from contaminated groundwater at a long-standing smelter site by precipitation as metal sulfides, yielding outflow metal concentrations below the parts per billion range (Barnes et al 1992).

Phosphatase-mediated metal precipitation. Metal or radionuclide accumulation by bacterial biomass is mediated by the activity of a phosphatase enzyme, induced during metal-free growth, that liberates inorganic phosphate from a supplied organic phosphate donor molecule. This then precipitates metal/radionuclide cations as phosphates on the biomass (Macaskie & Dean 1989). Most work has been carried out with a *Citrobacter* sp., and a range of bioreactor configurations have been described (Macaskie & Dean 1989, Tolley et al 1995).

Reduction. A promising application of dissimilatory biological metal reduction is uranium precipitation and removal from solution. This may have potential both in waste treatment and in concentrating uranium from low-grade sources (Lovley 1995). The reason is that while uranyl U(VI) compounds are readily soluble, U(IV) compounds such as the hydroxide or carbonate have low solubility and readily form precipitates at neutral pH. An iron-reducing organism (GS-15) can reduce U(VI) to U(IV) in a dissimilatory process with the U(IV) accumulating as a black precipitate in association with the bacterial cells (Lovley et al 1991). Sulfate-reducing bacteria can also carry out reduction of U(VI) to U(IV) and it has been suggested that this reaction is responsible for the observed high local concentrations of precipitated uranium in sediments under sulfate-reducing conditions (Lovley & Phillips 1992). The reduction kinetics of uranium(VI) in solution by *Desulphovibrio desulphuricans* was consistent with reduction coupled to bacterial growth, and could occur in the presence of sulfate. As this process produced a very pure precipitate of U(IV) carbonate, it was regarded as a viable alternative to removal by more conventional chemical technologies (Lovley & Phillips 1992, Lovley 1995).

High gradient magnetic separation. This is a technique for removal of metal ions from solution using bacteria rendered susceptible to magnetic fields. Precipitation of metal phosphates or sulfides on the surfaces of 'non-magnetic' bacteria is one of the methods that can make them magnetic (see Ellwood et al 1992).

Summary

Micro-organisms play important roles in the environmental fate of radionuclides in both aquatic and terrestrial ecosystems, with a multiplicity of physico-chemical and biological mechanisms effecting transformations between soluble and insoluble phases. Such mechanisms are important components of natural biogeochemical cycles for radionuclides and should be considered in any analyses of environmental radioactivity. In addition, several micro-organism-based biotechnologies, e.g. those based on biosorption or precipitation, are of potential use for the treatment of radionuclide contamination.

Acknowledgements

I am grateful for financial support from the Natural Environment Research Council/ Agricultural and Food Research Council (Special Topic Programme: Pollutant transport in soils and rocks), the Biotechnology and Biological Sciences Research Council (grant numbers: BCE 03292, SPC 2922, SPC 02812), the Royal Society (London) (638072:P779 Project grant), the Royal Society of Edinburgh (Scottish Office Education Department/RSE Support Research Fellowship 1994-1995) and the North Atlantic Treaty Organization (ENVIR.LG.950387 Linkage grant).

References

Avery SV 1995 Caesium accumulation by microorganisms: uptake mechanisms, cation competition, compartmentalization and toxicity. J Ind Microbiol 14:76–84
Avery SV 1996 Fate of caesium in the environment: distribution between the abiotic and biotic components of aquatic and terrestrial ecosystems. J Environ Radioact 30:139–171
Avery SV, Codd GA, Gadd GM 1992 Interactions of cyanobacteria and microalgae with caesium. In: Vernet J-P (ed) Impact of heavy metals on the environment. Elsevier, Amsterdam, p 133–182
Barnes LJ, Janssen FJ, Scheeren PJM, Versteegh JH, Koch RO 1992 Simultaneous microbial removal of sulphate and heavy metals from wastewater. Trans Inst Mining Metall 101:183–189
Beveridge TJ, Doyle RJ 1989 Metal ions and bacteria. Wiley, New York
Birch L, Bachofen R 1990 Complexing agents from microorganisms. Experientia 46:827–834
Brierley CL 1990 Bioremediation of metal-contaminated surface and groundwaters. Geomicrobiol J 8:201–223

Brierley CL, Brierley JA, Davidson MS 1989 Applied microbial processes for metals recovery and removal from wastewater. In: Beveridge TJ, Doyle RJ (eds) Metal ions and bacteria. Wiley, New York, p 359–382

de Rome L, Gadd GM 1991 Use of pelleted and immobilized yeast and fungal biomass for heavy metal and radionuclide recovery. J Industrial Microbiol 7:97–104

Dighton J, Terry G 1996 Uptake and immobilization of caesium in UK grassland and forest soils by fungi, following the Chernobyl accident. In: Frankland JC, Magan N, Gadd GM (eds) Fungi and environmental change. Cambridge University Press, Cambridge, p 184–200

Ellwood DC, Hill MJ, Watson JHP 1992 Pollution control using microorganisms and magnetic separation. In: Fry JC, Gadd GM, Herbert RA, Jones CW, Watson-Craik I (eds) Microbial control of pollution. Cambridge University Press, Cambridge, p 89–112

Fortin D, Davis B, Southam G, Beveridge TJ 1995 Biogeochemical phenomena induced by bacteria within sulphidic mine tailings. J Industrial Microbiol 14:178–185

Francis AJ 1990 Microbial dissolution and stabilization of toxic metals and radionuclides in mixed wastes. Experientia 46:840–851

Francis AJ 1994 Microbial transformations of radioactive wastes and environmental restoration through bioremediation. J Alloys Compounds 213:226–231

Francis AJ, Dodge CJ, Gillow JB 1992 Biodegradation of metal citrate complexes and implications for toxic-metal mobility. Nature 356:140–142

Gadd GM 1988 Accumulation of metals by microorganisms and algae. In: Rehm H-J (ed) Biotechnology, vol 6b: Special microbial processes. VCH Verlagsgesellschaft, Weinheim, p 401-433

Gadd GM 1990 Fungi and yeasts for metal accumulation. In: Ehrlich H, Brierley CL (eds) Microbial mineral recovery. McGraw-Hill, New York, p 249–275

Gadd GM 1992 Microbial control of heavy metal pollution. In: Fry JC, Gadd GM, Herbert RA, Jones CW, Watson-Craik I (eds) Microbial control of pollution. Cambridge University Press, Cambridge, p 59–88

Gadd GM 1993a Interactions of fungi with toxic metals. New Phytol 124:25–60

Gadd GM 1993b Microbial formation and transformation of organometallic and organometalloid compounds. FEMS Microbiol Rev 11:297–316

Gadd GM, White C 1990 Biosorption of radionuclides by yeast and fungal biomass. J Chem Technol Biotechnol 49:331–343

Gadd GM, White C 1993 Microbial treatment of metal pollution — a working biotechnology? Trends Biotechnol 11:353–359

Landa ER, Gray JR 1995 US Geological Survey: research on the environmental fate of uranium mining and milling wastes. Environ Geol 26:19–31

Lovley DR 1993 Dissimilatory metal reduction. Ann Rev Microbiol 47:263–290

Lovley DR 1995 Bioremediation of organic and metal contaminants with dissimilatory metal reduction. J Industrial Microbiol 14:85–93

Lovley DR, Phillips EJP 1992 Reduction of uranium by *Desulphovibrio desulphuricans*. Appl Environ Microbiol 58:850–856

Lovley DR, Phillips EJP, Gorby YA, Landa ER 1991 Microbial reduction of uranium. Nature 350:413–416

Macaskie LE 1991 The application of biotechnology to the treatment of wastes produced from the nuclear fuel cycle: biodegradation and bioaccumulation as a means of treating radionuclide-containing streams. Crit Rev Biotechnol 11:41–112

Macaskie LE, Dean ACR 1989 Microbial metabolism, desolubilization, and deposition of heavy metals: uptake by immobilised cells and application to the treatment of liquid wastes. In: Mizrahi A (ed) Biological waste treatment. Liss Inc, New York, p 150–201

Macaskie LE, Dean ACR 1990 Metal-sequestering biochemicals. In: Volesky B (ed) Biosorption of heavy metals. CRC Press, Boca Raton, FL, p 199–248

Mehra RK, Winge DR 1991 Metal ion resistance in fungi: molecular mechanisms and their related expression. J Cell Biochem 45:30–40

Morley GF, Sayer JA, Wilkinson SC, Gharieb MM, Gadd GM 1996 Fungal sequestration, mobilization and transformation of metals and metalloids. In: Frankland JC, Magan N, Gadd GM (eds) Fungi and environmental change. Cambridge University Press, Cambridge, p 235–256

Perkins J, Gadd GM 1995 The influence of pH and external K^+ concentration on caesium toxicity and accumulation in *Escherichia coli* and *Bacillus subtilis*. J Industrial Microbiol 14:218–225

Rusin PA, Quintana L, Brainard JR et al 1994 Solubilization of plutonium hydrous oxide by iron-reducing bacteria. Environ Sci Technol 28:1686–1690

Tobin J, White C, Gadd GM 1994 Fungal accumulation of toxic metals and application to environmental technology. J Industrial Microbiol 13:126–130

Tolley MR, Strachan LF, Macaskie LM 1995 Lanthanum accumulation from acidic solutions using a *Citrobacter* sp. immobilized in a flow-through bioreactor. J Industrial Microbiol 14:271–280

Volesky B (ed) 1990 Biosorption of heavy metals. CRC Press, Boca Raton, FL

White C, Wilkinson SC, Gadd GM 1995 The role of microorganisms in biosorption of toxic metals and radionuclides. Int Biodet Biodeg 35:17–40

DISCUSSION

Voigt: You have shown us how bacteria can remove caesium, for example, from solutions, but is the application of bacteria as a countermeasure in the open field realistic?

Gadd: Most of the conventional treatment methods for caesium rely on physical or chemical methods and a biological treatment method for caesium treatment in the field is probably unrealistic. Avery et al (1993) have proposed one treatment whereby a salt-tolerant alga, *Chlorella salina*, is stimulated by high salinity to take up large quantities of caesium from solution when grown in laboratory bioreactors. However, there would be problems with applying this in the field unless it was for the treatment of caesium-contaminated effluent or waste water. In terms of the remediation of the terrestrial environment, introduction of such micro-organisms may not be such a good idea because the environment would be disturbed further. However, there are many examples of microbial methods being used for the clean-up of toxic metals from aqueous wastes and some of these are now being applied to terrestrial systems (see Gadd 1992). Caesium, on the other hand, is more problematic because it is very mobile and does not form many insoluble precipitates in the same way that copper or cadmium, for example, do. There is a project in operation in Holland (the Shell–Budelco process) that uses sulfate-reducing bacteria to precipitate toxic metals, mainly zinc, in the waste as insoluble sulfides. This is a good example of recycling because there is a lot of zinc sulfate at the smelter site which goes into the reactor. The bacteria reduce the sulfate, producing hydrogen sulfide, and the zinc is precipitated as sulfide and reused in the smelting process. This has been in operation since about 1992 (Barnes et al 1992). Many other schemes have been devised for waste streams, based on biosorptive technologies with freely suspended cells, immobilized cells and biofilms on different matrices, although many of these processes have not been used on a commercial scale (Gadd & White 1993, White et al 1995).

We have been involved in a project with British Nuclear Fuels PLC and Viridian Bioprocessing to look at the detoxification of polluted wastes and effluents. We have been examining the possibility of using sulfur-oxidizing bacteria, such as *Thiobacillus* sp., to leach metals from contaminated soil in a bioreactor, although this approach may be too complex for *in situ* application. The *Thiobacillus* produces an acidic leachate that contains the metals, which could include uranium. The leachate is then passed into a sulfate-reducing bacterial bioreactor which precipitates the metals as sulfides. Disposal of the sulfidic sludge depends on a number of factors, but a biomineralization procedure has been proposed that would involve treating the sulfide to form a stable vitreous product that could be stored.

Håkanson: I have participated in two projects dealing with countermeasures in nature. Liming, fertilization and potash treatments have been tested in lakes, but none of them are very cost-effective. Could you give us some advice about the practical use of ecologically relevant countermeasures that are cost-effective?

Gadd: There are some examples that involve mining leachates, which could presumably be applied to radionuclides (see Gadd 1992, Gadd & White 1993, White et al 1995). For example, there are some mining areas in Missouri that had dilute leachates and wastes coming out into the water. One system that was used to treat this was to set up lagoons where algal growth was encouraged. The algal blooms can remove some metals by biosorption and when they eventually die, decay of the biomass results in anaerobic conditions and metal immobilization as sulfides. Some of these processes have apparently worked so well that the treated water has been used to supply a fish farm.

There are other good examples that involve methylation, although this process may not be feasible for radionuclides in the field. Methylation has been used most successfully for selenium. Selenium derivatives contaminated a large area in California, i.e. the Kesterson reservoir in the San Joaquin valley. This was natural pollution arising from weathering of seleniferous deposits, and ultimately leading to teratogenic effects in birds breeding in this wet-land. The clean-up of this was simple and apparently cost-effective. Lagoons were drained to produce selenium-rich sediments, to which was added waste organic material. Indigenous micro-organisms were stimulated to grow and these methylated virtually all of the selenium over a two-year period (see Thompson-Eagle & Frankenberger 1992). The cost-effective nature of some of these microbial processes was one of the main reasons why they were proposed in the first place.

In addition, I should point out that because some of the more traditional countermeasures for metal/radionuclide detoxification are not completely 100% effective, it has been proposed that some microbial processes may be used as a polisher to physico-chemical treatments, rather than be complete replacements of them (Gadd 1992).

Konoplev: Do you know of any quantitative measurements of caesium selectivity in terms of the ion-exchange mechanisms on the cell wall and cell membrane? Also, is it possible in the field to predict the rates of transformation processes of radionuclides or heavy metals on the basis of the micro-organism status of the soil, for example, in terms of rate constants?

Gadd: In answer to your first question, in microbial biomass caesium and other related monovalent metal cations, e.g. Na^+ and K^+, have a low affinity in terms of ion exchange: almost any other metal cation can replace them. Negligible amounts may be associated with the cell walls in fungi, algae and bacteria, although there are some exceptions, which include organisms with certain pigments that seem to bind more caesium than non-pigmented organisms. The majority of caesium accumulated in cells appears to be via active transport across the plasma membrane (Avery et al 1991, 1993, Gadd & White 1993, Perkins & Gadd 1996).

Secondly, it is generally accepted, except in the most simple of situations, that predictions of metal/radionuclide transformation rates in the soil in relation to microbial status are difficult, if not impossible. This problem is manifest because of the great complexity of the soil environment. It could be assumed, however, that in certain soil environments one would be able to identify a particular microbial activity which would be of importance. For example, in a black, anaerobic sediment one would be able to identify metal sulfide precipitation as an important process mediated by sulfate-reducing bacteria. Also, in some acidic forest soils fungi are responsible for much of the caesium accumulation. However, in general it is extremely difficult to determine different rates and their relative importance within a complex terrestrial environment where physico-chemical and biological processes are important.

Aarkrog: As far as I understood, you implied that bacteria could act in a similar fashion to ion exchangers and that in order to compete with ion exchangers one should be able to absorb 15% of the bacterial weight of ^{137}Cs, for example. In this case, the amount of ^{137}Cs activity in a bacterial population of 1 kg, would be in the order of 0.5 pBq. Although bacteria are resistant to irradiation, I could imagine that there would be problems with such a high concentration of radioactivity in the bacterial population. How much radioactivity can bacteria tolerate?

Gadd: As I explained previously, the use of micro-organisms as ion exchangers for caesium is unfeasible because of their low affinity for caesium; the 15% value is taken from work concerned with the recovery of other metals, including precious metals (see Gadd 1992). Regarding your comment about sensitivity of microbes to irradiation, I am not entirely sure of the answer as I do not work on this specific aspect. However, although little work has been carried out, I do know that there are some incredibly resistant bacteria. There are even bacteria, e.g. *Micrococcus radiodurans*, that can be isolated from soil proximal to atomic blasts.

Frissel: I would like to add a few points on the role of micro-organisms in radioecology; not so much on specific actions, such as those that Geoffrey Gadd has described, but on the effects of normal microbiological processes. Micro-organisms require at least carbon, nitrogen and oxygen for growth. To obtain the carbon, they decompose the soil organic matter using oxygen. The source of the oxygen is atmospheric oxygen, which diffuses into the soil. If a soil becomes waterlogged, the diffusion is hampered and oxygen becomes depleted. The micro-organisms will then use other sources with a high redox potential to maintain their growth, e.g. iron oxides and manganese oxides. The result is a decrease of the adsorption sites in a soil, which may result in increased leaching. A second consequence is that a decreasing redox potential influences the chemical status of many radionuclides, including plutonium, americium, iodine and technetium. For example, it is often stated that technetium is present as a very mobile ion, but this is only the case at high redox potentials; at low redox potentials, it is completely reduced and almost completely adsorbed. A third consequence is that metal ions and other ions may be methylated. From a radioecological point of view, the methylation of iodine is important, although the most important methylation product may be methyl mercury, which is usually not radioactive. A fourth result is that the nitrogen cycle changes. The normal process is that during decomposition of organic matter, if the carbon/nitrogen quotient of the organic matter is sufficiently low, ammonium is formed, which may be oxidized to nitrate and subsequently denitrified. In cold, waterlogged soils, however, ammonium is stable and oxidation to nitrate does not occur. The result is that the ammonium ions compete with the caesium ions for adsorption sites. This is one of the reasons why caesium in upland soils — and this concerns upland soils that are relatively cold and boggy — is more available for root uptake than in normal agricultural soils.

There is another microbiological process involving nitrogen that is important. In pastures which are never fertilized the proportion of plants that practice symbiotic nitrogen fixation is rather large. Such plants have an ecological advantage over other plants. If nitrogen fertilizers are applied this advantage disappears, and consequently the proportion of nitrogen-fixing plants decreases. The most abundant nitrogen-fixing plants include *Trifolium hybridum* L. and *Trifolium pratense* L., which have transfer factors of 5.0 and 8.1 m^2/kg, respectively. The most abundant non-nitrogen-fixing plants in modern pastures include *Poa pratense* L. *and Phleum pratense* L., which have transfer factors of 0.6 and 0.7 m^2/kg, respectively. By suppressing the symbiotic nitrogen fixation it is therefore possible to reduce the uptake of caesium on a pasture considerably. This has been successfully applied in the former Soviet Union.

Konoplev: I have a small remark concerning the transfer factors after the Chernobyl accident. During the first few years after the accident, high transfer factors were observed because of surface contamination by atmospheric fallout and resuspension. This process does not involve root uptake.

Frissel: It does involve root uptake: after one year uptake via leaves was negligible compared to root uptake. A consideration of resuspension and rain splash is important, certainly in the case of caesium, because about 50% of the uptake is caused by rain splash.

Streffer: What exactly do you mean by the term 'rain splash'?

Frissel: Rain splash indicates that the crop is contaminated with soil which splashes up due to the impact of raindrops when they hit the soil surface. This process involves relatively heavy soil particles. It is not equivalent to the term resuspension, which, in my opinion, should be used for relatively light particles that may be transported via air over longer distance. By contrast, rain splash has only short-range effects.

Howard: This is really a term for soil adhesion or mass loading, and one has to be careful because it can be extremely variable, i.e. it can vary from less than a few per cent of the biomass of vegetation to over 30%. The importance of soil also varies according to the amount of root uptake versus the amount in the soil. Therefore, the concept of soil adhesion is important, but it's extremely variable depending on the radionuclide mobility, pasture type and the weather, for example.

Frissel: I agree. However, for plutonium and americium rain splash and soil adhesion dominate over root uptake, whereas for caesium root uptake and soil adhesion are roughly equal. For strontium, the root uptake dominates. We have to accept that there is a high level of uncertainty in these situations.

Howard: The dominance of root uptake is probably true for any mobile radionuclide, except for situations of very low vegetation biomass or special conditions such as external contamination of vegetation surfaces.

Gadd: Rain splash and other aerial depositions are also responsible for confusion over the levels of caesium in fungal fruiting bodies. There is often an inadequate distinction between translocation of caesium along the hyphae to the fruit bodies and that which becomes associated with the fruit bodies by aerial deposition (see Gadd & White 1993). Some of this confusion may be caused by lack of care in analysis.

References

Avery SV, Codd GA, Gadd GM 1991 Caesium accumulation and interactions with other monovalent cations in the cyanobacterium *Synechocystis* PCC 6803. J Gen Microbiol 137:405–413

Avery SV, Codd GA, Gadd GM 1993 Salt stimulation of caesium accumulation by *Chlorella salina*: potential relevance to the development of a biological Cs-removal process. J Gen Microbiol 139:2239–2244

Barnes LJ, Janssen FJ, Scheeren PJM, Versteegh JH, Koch RO 1992 Simultaneous microbial removal of sulphate and heavy metals from wastewater. Trans Inst Mining Metall 101:183–189

Gadd GM 1992 Microbial control of heavy metal pollution. In: Fry JC, Gadd GM, Herbert RA, Jones CW, Watson-Craik I (eds) Microbial control of pollution. Cambridge University Press, Cambridge, p 59–88

Gadd GM, White C 1993 Microbial treatment of metal pollution — a working biotechnology? Trends Biotechnol 11:353–359

Perkins J, Gadd GM 1996 Interactions of Cs^+ and other monovalent cations (Li^+, Na^+, Rb^+, NH_4^+) with K^+-dependent pyruvate kinase and malate dehydrogenase from the yeasts *Rhodotorula rubra* and *Saccharomyces cerevisiae*. Mycol Res 100:449–454

Thompson-Eagle ET, Frankenberger WT 1992 Bioremediation of soils contaminated with selenium. In: Lal R, Stewart BA (eds) Advances in Soil Science, vol 17. Springer, New York, p 261–309

White C, Wilkinson SC, Gadd GM 1995 The role of microorganisms in biosorption of toxic metals and radionuclides. Int Biodet Biodeg 35:17–40

The fate and impact of radiocontaminants in urban areas

Jørn Roed, Kasper G. Andersson and Christian Lange

Contamination Physics Group, Environmental Science and Technology Department, Risø National Laboratory, PO Box 49, DK-4000 Roskilde, Denmark

Abstract. The Chernobyl accident made it clear that the contaminants released after a severe nuclear accident may spread over large areas, and thereby form a significant external radiation hazard in areas of high population density. Since then, the weathering effects on the deposited radiocontaminants (essentially radiocaesium) have been followed on different types of surface in urban, suburban and industrial areas in order to enable an estimation of the long-term impact of such events. Analytical expressions have been derived for the typical behaviour of radiocaesium on the different surfaces, and dose measurements and calculations for different urban environments have pinpointed which surfaces generally contribute most to the dose and consequently are most important to clean. At this point, after nearly a decade, the dose rate from horizontal pavements has decreased by at least a factor of 10, whereas the dose rate from an area of soil or a roof has generally only been halved. The contamination on walls is the most persistent: it has only decreased by 10–20 %.

1997 Health impacts of large releases of radionuclides. Wiley, Chichester (Ciba Foundation Symposium 203) p 109–119

One main purpose of investigating a contaminated urban environment is to estimate the health burden to the population in terms of the dose received in the area over a period of time. In order to make an adequate estimate of doses received in the past, or indeed in the future, it is imperative to know not only the initial contaminant concentrations, but also how the levels of contamination on the different surfaces in an urban environment will change due to weathering effects over variable periods of time. Where this natural dose reduction is insufficient to restore the area at least to the recommended maximum levels, forced decontamination may be the solution.

Radiocaesium deposition in urban areas

The most important radionuclide concerning the long-term external dose in inhabited areas is ^{137}Cs. In general, airborne radiopollutants take the form of either liquid drops, reactive or inert gases, and aerosols (including larger fragments). Airborne radiopollutants can be depleted from the air by various processes that lead to

TABLE 1   Relative source strengths for various surfaces shortly after deposition of Chernobyl fallout caesium, relative to that on a cut lawn (1.00), where there is no penetration into the soil

Surface	Dry deposition	Wet deposition
Gardens, parks	1.00	0.80
Roofs	1.00	0.40
Walls	0.10	0.01
Streets, pavements	0.40	0.50
Trees with leaves	3.00	0.10

deposition. If precipitation is present the process is termed wet deposition (and dry deposition in the absence of precipitation). Variations can occur within these different categories of deposition; for example, the deposition pattern resulting from a light rain shower gives little surface run-off compared with that resulting from prolonged heavy rain.

A series of measurements by Roed (1990) of radiocaesium dry deposition in Danish urban areas after the Chernobyl accident in 1986 revealed that the deposition velocities (ratio of the air concentration at 1 m above the surface to the dry deposition flux to the surface) were small compared with those found for rural areas at comparable distances from the accident site. The measured deposition velocities (in 10^{-4} m/s) on paved areas, walls, windows, grass (clipped), trees and roofs were 0.7, 0.1, 0.05, 4.3, 7 and 2.8, respectively. Estimates by Roed (1990), based on measurements of Chernobyl fallout in areas that received only dry deposition and those in which deposition took place with heavy rain, revealed the typical relationships between caesium contamination levels per unit area of different types of surface (Table 1). A comparison showed the figures to be consistent with those obtained by measurements made in various parts of Europe. The factor of 0.80 rather than 1.00 for wet deposition in soil areas is explained by the slight penetration of the isotopes into the soil giving a shielding factor of 0.80.

Measurements of radiocaesium weathering in housing environments

After the initial interception of deposited contamination by a surface, the surface is exposed to weathering processes — such as wind, frost, precipitation and mechanical impact — that deplete the adsorbed radioactive matter. The influence of human activities, such as traffic and routine street cleaning, is often also interpreted as contributing to weathering because it is difficult to distinguish the different processes leading to the reduction of contamination.

Since the Chernobyl accident, the weathering effects on different types of surface in urban, suburban and industrial areas have been followed through six measurement campaigns in the Gävle area in Sweden, which received high levels of contamination following heavy rain shortly after the accident. The radiocaesium levels were measured on various surfaces, including walls, grassed areas, pavements, walkways and roads (Table 2). Although the first campaign was made in 1987, a comparison with other measurements made in the same area in May 1986 to October 1986 (Karlberg & Sundblad 1986) made it possible to relate the measured results to the initial radiocaesium deposition in the area.

The dose rate reductions that were recorded in Gävle on grassed areas were dependent on the soil type, and several different vertical distribution profiles of ^{137}Cs have been recorded. During the first 8.5 years following deposition, the dose rate from areas of soil decreased by 40–60%. However, there was little, if any, decrease in the levels of radiocaesium contamination on walls of buildings over the same period. Indeed, in one measurement (a wall of the Gevalia building in 1993) the level actually increased. This increase is, however, not highly significant, and it could be caused by a wash-down of radioactive substances from the upper parts of the wall. A measurement at this site the following year showed the expected decrease. A yellow brick wall of the fire station had a low level of contamination compared with the other walls because it was exposed only to dry deposition (the structure of the building protects the wall from precipitation).

In contrast to the situation on walls, the levels of radiocaesium on asphalt surfaces have decreased to 10% of the level measured in 1988. A comparison with the results of Karlberg & Sundblad (1986) indicates that less than 2% of the initially deposited radiocaesium now remains on the road. The levels on these surfaces are now below the detection limit. This finding is in agreement with previous laboratory investigations, which have shown that only a small fraction of radiocaesium contamination is associated with the bitumen in the asphalt, and that a greater proportion is associated with a thin layer of street dust, which will eventually be subjected to weathering.

Measurements made in 1993 in Pripyat (near the Chernobyl reactor) showed higher residual levels of radiocaesium on roads, but this town was evacuated early, and there has been a limited amount of traffic on the roads since the contamination. The radiocaesium on the different surfaces in Pripyat was, however, easier to remove than in Gävle. Two possible explanations for this may be envisaged: that the loosely held part of the contamination had not been removed by human activity; and that the deposition in Pripyat involved large (insoluble) core fragment particles.

Ten per cent of the initially deposited radiocaesium remains on paved concrete surfaces. No significant decrease has been recorded over the last three years, suggesting that the radiocaesium is firmly fixed. Weathering on horizontal hard surfaces generally occurred more rapidly in the more heavily trafficked spots.

The contamination levels of clay roof tiles, initially contaminated by the Chernobyl accident and exposed to weathering processes in Gävle for four years, have been

TABLE 2 ^{137}Cs levels measured in Gävle, Sweden in 1987, 1988, 1990, 1991, 1993 and 1994

Location	Surface	Material	Orientation	^{137}Cs levels measured in Gävle, Sweden[a] (kBq/m^2)					
				1987	1988	1990	1991	1993	1994
City hall	Wall	Plaster	South-east	—	0.78±11%	—	—	—	0.53±12%
City hall	Wall	Plaster	South-west	—	0.55±16%	—	—	—	0.21±27%
City hall	Paving	Flagstone[b]	Middle[b]	—	9.71±6%	4.26±7%	3.13±8%	3.10±9%	—
City hall	Paving	Flagstone	West	—	6.40±6%	3.15±6%	2.17±8%	2.12±9%	2.12±6%
City hall	Road	Asphalt		—	1.49±9%	0.44±17%	—	—	—
Gevalia company	Wall	Red brick	South, washing	1.93±9%	1.65±9%	—	—	—	—
Gevalia company	Wall	Red brick	North, washing	—	3.93±7%	—	1.85±7%	2.13±15%	1.89±7%
Fire station	Wall	Yellow brick	North, dry deposition	—	0.42±15%	—	—	—	0.14±36%
Transformer substation	Wall	Yellow brick	South, washing	—	1.06±11%	—	0.80±10%	—	—
Magasin Street	Wall	Plaster	North, washing	0.99±10%	—	—	0.98±10%	0.76±10%	—
General Foods company	Wall	Plaster	East	—	1.14±10%	—	—	—	0.59±12%
Fire station	Paving	Asphalt and flagstone		—	—	3.21±8%	2.38±8%	—	—
Gevalia	Car park	Asphalt		3.17±7%	3.28±7%	—	—	—	—
Gevalia	Crossroads	Asphalt		—	1.19±9%	—	—	—	—

[a]Measurement ± uncertainty corresponding to 2 S.D.
[b]Middle part of flagstone paving in front of city hall.

TABLE 3   **Typical weathering parameter values of various types of urban surface**

	Slow component		Fast component	
Surface	Fraction	Half-life (days)	Fraction	Half-life (days)
Roofs	0.7	7.0×10^3	0.3	3.5×10^2
Pavings	0.5	7.0×10^2	0.5	7.0×10^1
Walls	0.9	2.0×10^4	0.1	7.0×10^1

measured in Risø. These tiles were subsequently exposed to Danish weather on a specially constructed scaffold, and a decrease in the radiocaesium contamination level ranging from 28 to 35% was measured over the following 19 months. This is in reasonably good agreement with other measurements at Risø on different types of roof contaminated by Chernobyl fallout.

Weathering processes affecting roofs, walls and horizontal pavings have a slow and a fast component, and can be adequately described over the first decade by two-component exponential functions. Some typical values of the parameters are given in Table 3.

In conclusion, weathering processes do not sufficiently reduce the contamination levels on many important urban surfaces, even over a 10-year period. Therefore, forced decontamination may be called for in areas of high levels of contamination.

Decontamination of housing environments

Since the Chernobyl accident, many methods have been investigated for the decontamination of the heavily contaminated areas of the former Soviet Union. Small- and large-scale experiments have been conducted (e.g. Roed 1990, 1991, Roed & Andersson 1996) and, based on recent medium-scale investigations, parameters regarding the individual practicable methods have been derived (Roed et al 1995). Strategies based on these investigations, together with computer models, have been suggested for the decontamination of different types of housing environments (Andersson et al 1995). In general, computer modelling has demonstrated that soil areas contribute the largest dose, although other surfaces are also important, depending on the type of environment.

The methods found to be the most cost-effective were subjected to large-scale tests in a settlement at Novo Bobovitsi in Russia in the late summer of 1995. This work, which was supported by the Danish Ministry of the Interior, was unique in the sense that it was the first project to investigate the full effect, under field conditions, of a whole decontamination strategy consisting mainly of countermeasures developed/adapted by the Commission of the European Communities Experimental Collaboration Project no. 4 (ECP/4) international group of experts. The effect of each sequence in the strategy was recorded in terms of contamination removal/translocation and dose rate reduction at various reference points indoors and outdoors. Monitoring the contamination levels on the different surfaces in the environment revealed that the main contributors to the dose rate were the soil areas and roofs of the buildings. The relative contribution from the latter was found to be greater than that found in most previously investigated areas. For the decontamination of roofs, a special roof-cleaning device was applied (Roed & Andersson 1996), and from the garden areas around the buildings, soil was removed to a depth of 6–7 cm. Subsequent to the soil removal, a 4 cm layer of gravel was applied to the decontaminated surface to shield against the residual radiation from radiocaesium that had penetrated beyond the depth of the removed soil layer. A contaminated layer of pine needles was removed from the roofs with a rake prior to the actual roof decontamination. Figure 1 shows the relative reductions, inside three of the decontaminated houses, of the dose rate for the different steps of the strategy. On Houses 4 and 5 the roof was cleaned using the special roof-cleaning device, but the roof of House 6 was removed and replaced.

This strategy resulted in a reduced dose rate due to Chernobyl fallout by up to 64%. This percentage can be taken as a minimum, because much larger areas would be decontaminated if a political decision were made to apply the strategy in reality. It can also be seen that the residual dose rate is greatest in House 4, which is closest to untreated areas, and smallest in House 6, which is surrounded by decontaminated soil and shielded by neighbouring walls.

Calculations based on other measurements have shown that contaminated indoor surfaces may, under some circumstances (i.e. dry deposition), contribute almost as much to the total dose as outdoor surfaces (Andersson et al 1995). In Novo Bobovitsi, however, outdoor contamination occurred as a result of precipitation, and the dose contributions from deposition on walls (outdoor or indoor) were small. Indoor contamination may have resulted from the accidental introduction of outdoor contamination (e.g. on the soles of people's shoes) inside houses (where people spend about 85% of their time).

Another countermeasure that was tested at Novo Bobovitsi was the triple-digging procedure. The principle of this procedure is visualized in Fig. 2. Only a relatively thin layer containing all the contamination is buried in the bottom of the soil depth profile. The thickness of this layer can be adjusted according to the contamination penetration depth. The thin top soil layer is inverted, but the soil from the lower layers is not inverted; thereby, the impact on the soil fertility and on the future crop production is minimized. The area tested by this procedure at Novo Bobovitsi measured 10 m × 10 m.

This procedure reduced the external dose rate by a factor of 2.1, which is in good agreement with the predictions of Monte Carlo simulations based on soil profile samples. These calculations, however, also showed that if an area of 100 m × 100m or more had been treated (as would have been done in practice if the political decision had been made to clean the area), the external dose would have been reduced by a factor of

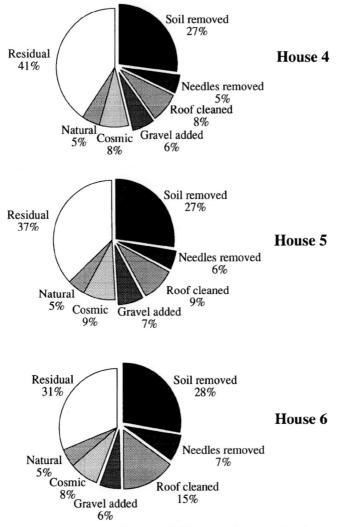

FIG. 1.   Pie charts showing the contributions of different environmental surfaces to the dose rate inside three different houses at Novo Bobovitsi. The effects of different cleaning operations are indicated. After the operation, a cosmic, a natural and a residual fallout fraction remain.

at least 10. A detailed report of the work in Novo Bobovitsi can be found in Roed et al (1996).

Conclusions

The long-term weathering effects on urban surfaces contaminated with ^{137}Cs have been examined in six field campaigns in Sweden and measurements in the former Soviet

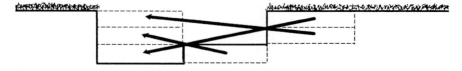

FIG. 2.   Diagrammatic representation of the triple-digging procedure showing how the order of the three soil layers is changed. The total depth of digging at Novo Bobovitsi was 30 cm.

Union. Weathering effects on road pavings, walls and roofs can be adequately described over the first decade by two-component exponential functions. The roofs and soil areas have retained much of the deposited radiocaesium, even after almost a decade. Nine years after the Chernobyl accident, large-scale experiments have been conducted in a Russian settlement to investigate the effect on the whole environment of the introduction of a strategy based on cost-effective countermeasures for these types of surface. It was found that the dose rate inside a house could be reduced by two-thirds. If a larger area were treated, the dose reduction could be much greater: possibly by a factor of 10.

Acknowledgements

This work was partially funded by the commission of the European Communities under the Radiation Protection Programme and by the Danish Emergency Management Agency.

References

Andersson KG, Roed J, Roed J, Paretzke HG, Tschiesch J 1995 Modelling of the radiological impact of a deposit of artificial radionuclides in inhabited areas. In: Deposition of radionuclides, their subsequent relocation in the environment and resulting implications. CEC report EUR 16604 EN. European Commission, Brussels, p 83–94

Karlberg O, Sundblad B 1986 A Study of Weathering Effects on Deposited Activity in the Studsvik and Gävle Area. Studsvik Energite AB, S-611 82 Nyköping, Sweden

Roed J 1990 Deposition and removal of radioactive substances in an urban area. Nordic Liaison Committee for Atomic Energy. Final report of the NKA project AKTU-245. NORD 1990:111

Roed J 1991 Chapter 7 In: Sinnaeve J, Olast M (eds) Improvement of practical countermeasures: the urban environment. CEC Report EUR 12555 EN. European Commission, Brussels. p 190–233

Roed J, Andersson KG 1996 Clean-up of Urban Areas in the CIS Countries Contaminated by Chernobyl Fallout. J Environ Radioact 33:107–116

Roed J, Andersson KG, Prip H (eds) 1995 Practical means for decontamination 9 years after a nuclear accident. Risø-R-828(EN). Risø National Laboratory, Roskilde

Roed J, Lange C, Andersson KG et al 1996 Decontamination of a Russian settlement. Risø-R-870(EN). Risø National Laboratory, Roskilde

DISCUSSION

Konoplev: How long after the decontamination procedure were the effects of decontamination measured? The reason why I'm asking is that immediately after the accident some decontamination operations were carried out in the 30 km zone, and it was concluded that the efficiency of decontamination was low. It is possible that measurements taken immediately after the treatment indicate that decontamination has some effect, but that after a certain length of time there is little or no effect because of resuspension in the local area.

Roed: We have studied previous decontamination operations and we are also using models of resuspension so that we can predict the long-term dose reduction. We measured the effects 14 days after decontamination, but we have returned to these sites two or three years afterwards and shown that the decontamination procedure is still effective. We have demonstrated that it is possible to use these methods effectively over a large area.

Voigt: I have two questions. First, you showed us some data on roof tiles. Did you determine how far the different radionuclides penetrated into these tiles? Secondly, how high is the dose contribution to the person who is doing the triple digging?

Roed: The dose contribution to the person digging depends on the level of deposition. We are planning to decontaminate areas where people are living anyway, so the extra dose they receive from being out a little longer in their gardens would only be small.

In answer to your first question, we made some interesting measurements for radiocaesium, especially for radiocaesium contamination from bomb fallout. We found that the level of contamination was highest on the under side of the tiles. This is probably because heavy rain causes the diffusion of caesium ions through the tile, and when the top side dries up the transported caesium stays there. On the top side of the tile weathering processes will remove some of the deposited caesium, and after some time the contamination level on the under side may be higher than that at the top side. Therefore, it's not possible to decontaminate tiles efficiently if they are being polluted over a long period.

Balonov: I have a comment and a question. In 1989 in the area of Bryansk in Russia there was a large decontamination campaign undertaken by military groups under the supervision of radioprotection experts. We measured the effectiveness of this campaign throughout the following three to five years in different places, and we found that the dose rate levels were stable, i.e. the changes in dose rate over time were similar to those observed in non-decontaminated areas. The levels of resuspension over that time period were not significant because decontamination was carried out three years after the accident, but when decontamination was carried out immediately after the accident the resuspension rate was significant.

My question concerns the effectiveness of the decontamination. What was the decrease in annual dose received by people living in the houses?

Roed: We have not determined the external doses received by people in that area. Our goal was not to decontaminate a town, but to show how it could be done efficiently. It's up to the Russian government to do this. It's possible to calculate the dose reduction received by the people using dose rate measurements at the areas. In the future we should also look at the possibility of reducing doses received from consuming vegetables grown in gardens.

Renn: Have you ever considered planting special plants in the gardens that have the ability to concentrate radiocaesium, so that they could be harvested and disposed of at a later stage? Obviously, your triple-digging procedure does not remove the radiocaesium from the soil, it only covers the contaminated part by less-contaminated soil.

Roed: This has been looked at in the Experimental Collaboration Project no. 4 (ECP/ 4) of the International Scientific Collaboration on the consequences of the Chernobyl accident, which has been running over the last five years. Some scientists from Ukraine claim that it's possible to do it, but their evidence is not convincing and I don't believe that it can be done. We have to develop simple methods that can be used by everyone, and the triple-digging approach is one such method.

Paretzke: If an area is contaminated with 1 Bq radiocaesium per kg of soil, for example, and roots are growing at a depth of 20 cm, then the soil mass per m^2 is $240 \, kg/m^2$. Caesium has a high transfer factor, and if we assume that this is 1.0 then there would be 1 Bq/kg in fresh plants per 1 Bq/kg in the soil. If we further assume a normal biomass yield of $1 \, kg/m^2$ per year, then this would result in a decrease per year of 1 Bq out of the $204 \, Bq/m^2$. Therefore, it would take hundreds of years to remove the radiocaesium from the soil in this way.

Howard: I would like to pick up on the point that by decreasing the external dose you then become interested in the internal dose. The different sources of the ingestion dose have to be considered. For example, if these people have private cows, milk will be one of the most important internal sources, and if they also harvest from forests the relative intake from their vegetable plots will probably be low.

Roed: But in rural areas people do grow many vegetables in their gardens.

Howard: But the contribution of the vegetables to the internal radiocaesium intake is usually relatively small.

Roed: I would say it's about 25%.

Howard: It varies, depending on how much people use the forest and if they have a private cow or goat.

Streffer: What range of doses are we talking about?

Roed: The dose rate is more than 10 times that of the natural background rate—it's about 1200 nSv/h.

Paretzke: But the dose rate depends on many factors. In principle, if people live in a contaminated area and obtain all their food from this area, then they would receive about 50% of their total dose from external radiation and 50% from internal radiation.

Roed: And in the highly contaminated areas they would receive relatively more from external radiation because some of their food is obtained from less-contaminated areas.

Streffer: What is the annual dose in these areas?

Balonov: About 2 mSv.

Streffer: One has to consider whether this is cost-effective. There are many areas that have natural background radiation doses that are at least fivefold higher than this.

Roed: We have been working there for the last six to seven years, and we have the feeling that the people are ill, not necessarily because of the irradiation, but because of their anxiety. It seems that having people do something about their own situation, even if they only reduce their dose by a factor of two, has a positive psychological effect. It would be beneficial if psychologists talked to these people about the danger of irradiation and that it is not catastrophic to live here because they are afraid of living there.

Streffer: I am aware of all the psychological problems, but on the other hand we have to think about the permissible dose range. We may then be able to combine your programme with the psychological programmes to convince people that there are many areas that have higher dose rates. Also, it would be difficult to apply your method to agricultural land.

Roed: I disagree. It would be possible to reclaim agricultural land.

Streffer: But there would be a tremendous cost.

Roed: Not necessarily, we have developed a skim and burial plough, which can effectively carry out the triple-digging procedure in large areas, although it does take three times as much effort as a normal plough.

Paretzke: I would like to make a final comment in support of your work. Trying to reduce the total dose is often worthwhile, and reducing the external dose is sometimes easier than trying to reduce the internal dose.

Internal exposure of populations to long-lived radionuclides released into the environment

M. I. Balonov

Radioecology Department, Institute of Radiation Hygiene, Mira Street 8, 197101 St. Petersburg, Russia

Abstract. This chapter discusses the events that led to the contamination of environments with the long-lived radionuclides of caesium, strontium and other elements, and to the internal exposure of populations living in contaminated areas. Among these events are radioactive releases into the river Techa from the Soviet nuclear weapons facility Mayak in 1949–1956, thermonuclear weapons tests in the 1950s and 1960s, the Kyshtim and Windscale accidents in 1957, and the Chernobyl and Tomsk-7 accidents in 1986 and 1993, respectively. Methods of environmental monitoring and individual internal dose monitoring of inhabitants are described. These are based on measuring the content of radionuclides not only in the air, drinking water and local food products, but also in humans using whole-body counters and analysing excreta and autopsy samples. The dynamics of internal exposure of people of different ages to radionuclides of caesium, strontium and plutonium from the environment are considered. Examples of radionuclide distributions in the environment, and of individual/collective internal doses and related medical effects are presented.

1997 Health impacts of large releases of radionuclides. Wiley, Chichester (Ciba Foundation Symposium 203) p 120–138

The history of environmental contamination with man-made radionuclides in quantities that can have significant radiological consequences for populations goes back to the beginning of the nuclear industry in the USA, USSR and UK. Considerable amounts of radionuclides (mainly ^{131}I) were released into the atmosphere in 1944–1951 by the Hanford plant in northwest USA, and in 1948–1956 by the Mayak plant near Chelyabinsk (the Urals, USSR). In 1949–1952 liquid radioactive wastes of the Mayak plant containing long-lived ^{90}Sr and ^{137}Cs were released into the river Techa. Immediately after the production of nuclear weapons in the 1940s, the USA and USSR began testing them (and exploded two bombs above Japanese cities) in the atmosphere, on the ground surface, underwater and underground. These tests produced some local radioactive contamination of areas around test sites, but the bulk of long-lived radionuclides was released into the

TABLE 1 Major radioactive releases into the environment

Activity	Mode of release	
	Routine	Accidental
Military purposes		
weapons production	Hanford (1944–1951)	Techa river (1949–1951)
	Chelyabinsk (1948–1956)	Kyshtim (1957)
		Windscale (1957)
		Rocky Flats (1969)
		Tomsk-7 (1993)
atmospheric tests	Nevada (1951–1962)	Altay (1949)
	Semipalatinsk (1949–1962)	Marshall Islands (1954)
	Novaya Zemlya (1955–1962)	
nuclear fleet	Kola Peninsula	Chazhma (1985)
weapons transportation		Palomares (1966)
		Thule (1968)
Power production		
reactor operation	Worldwide	Three Mile Island (1979)
		Chernobyl (1986)
fuel processing	Sellafield	
	La Hague	
Radioisotope use		
loss of sources		Ciudad Juarez (1982)
		Goiania (1987)
satellite crash		SNAP-9A (1964, global)
		Cosmos-954 (1978, Canada)

stratosphere. These long-lived radionuclides were gradually deposited on the surface of the Earth, predominantly in the Northern hemisphere.

Subsequently, humans have used nuclear techniques even more widely. There are only five countries that legally produce nuclear weapons; however, 26 countries operate nuclear reactors, and radionuclides are applied in industry, medicine and science in most of the countries around the world. Releases of radionuclides into the environment have taken place mainly in the 1950s and 1960s, in connection with the nuclear arms race, nuclear technology imperfections and underestimations of the danger of radiation. Table 1 presents a classification of the regions that have been subjected to radioactive contaminations with man-made radionuclides (UNSCEAR 1993).

The variety of the sources and conditions of the releases, and of their consequent transport, causes different isotopic and physico-chemical compositions, and levels of radioactive contamination of the environment. Table 2 gives estimates for the releases of some of the fission products for major radiation events over the past five decades (UNSCEAR 1982, 1993, Nikipelov et al 1989, Iljin et al 1995). It is evident that the greatest amounts of radionuclides were released into the environment as a result of a series of high power nuclear tests in the atmosphere, mainly in 1957–1958 and 1961–1962. Long-term environmental contamination and population exposure remain in areas where there have been accidents at nuclear reactors (Chernobyl, Windscale) and releases from radioactive waste stores at the Mayak plant into the river Techa and in the atmosphere (Kyshtim).

Usually, the products of nuclear fission and neutron activation with half-lives over a year—namely, ^{3}H, ^{14}C, ^{90}Sr, ^{134}Cs, ^{137}Cs, plutonium isotopes and ^{241}Am—are classified as long-lived, man-made radionuclides that contaminate the environment. The soft beta emitters ^{3}H and ^{14}C are isotopes of the earth's macroelements and of its biosphere. Due to volatility of their main forms—^{3}H$_2$O and ^{14}CO$_2$—they can travel long distances before they decay. In this connection, they are classified as the so-called 'globally distributed' radionuclides, with their corresponding migration laws. In contrast, ^{90}Sr, ^{134}Cs, ^{137}Cs and plutonium isotopes do not travel widely and produce mainly local radiation effects, depending on local natural and climatic conditions. This chapter will only describe the consequences of environmental contamination with the latter group of radionuclides, and it will not discuss the behaviour of globally distributed ^{3}H and ^{14}C.

Radiological properties of strontium 90, caesium 137 and isotopes of plutonium

Strontium 90

^{90}Sr is an isotope of an element that belongs to the alkali earth group and is a chemical analogue of calcium. Its half-life is 29 years and it emits beta radiation with an average

TABLE 2   Releases of some important radionuclides into the environment (PBq)

Event	^{131}I	^{137}Cs	^{90}Sr	^{106}Ru	^{144}Ce	$^{239,240}Pu$
River Techa, 1949–1951		12	12	10–20	about 10	
Nuclear tests, 1952–1962	6.5×10^5	910	600	1.2×10^4	3.0×10^4	11
Kyshtim, 1957		0.03	2	1.4	24	
Windscale, 1957	0.7	0.02		0.003		
Karachay, 1967		0.01	0.004		0.004	
Chernobyl, 1986	1200	85	8	30	140	0.07
Goiania, 1987		0.05				
Tomsk-7, 1993				0.01	2×10^{-4}	6×10^{-6}

energy of 0.2 MeV. Its daughter radionuclide is ^{90}Y, which has a half-life of 2.7 days and emits beta radiation with an average energy of 0.9 MeV.

^{90}Sr migrates downward in virgin soil by diffusion and convective transport with a linear velocity at the migration front of about 0.2–0.4 cm/year. According to the data of Romanov et al (1990) obtained on the trace of the Kyshtim accident, the period of elimination of ^{90}Sr from the 2 cm layer of leached black earth is about five years, and from turf podzolic soil it is about two years. Moistening of the soil promotes migration because of the high solubility of strontium compounds. The surface water flow, mainly in spring, carries about 0.2% of ^{90}Sr activity per year.

The contamination of vegetation by aerogenic ^{90}Sr deposition on the surface of plants is dependent on foliage development and the conditions of the deposition (dry or wet). In a moderate climate, the specific activities of contaminated plants, which are influenced by precipitation, wind and the growth of plants, decrease exponentially with an average half life of about two weeks. Further, ^{90}Sr enters plants slowly through root systems and via secondary surface contamination caused by wind resuspension of soil particles. Plants in soils with high contents of clay, humus and calcium incorporate ^{90}Sr into their roots to a lesser extent than those from sandy soils. There can be up to 10–50-fold differences among the transfer factors of plants in different soils. About 0.1% of the ^{90}Sr absorbed by cows during a day is transferred to a litre of its milk, and there is an insignificant amount of ^{90}Sr in forest food products (such as mushrooms, berries and game meat). On average, 30% of ^{90}Sr activity is absorbed from the human intestinal tract into the bloodstream, and it accumulates in bone tissue of humans and animals. Since ^{90}Sr and ^{90}Y do not emit gamma radiation, their external action on humans is insignificant. Table 3 (ICRP 1993) presents the ^{90}Sr ingestion dose coefficients for different age groups. The dose coefficients are significantly higher for children and teenagers, reflecting calcium and strontium deposition during the formation of the skeleton.

Caesium 134 and 137

^{134}Cs and ^{137}Cs are radioactive isotopes of an element that belongs to the alkali group and is a chemical analogue of potassium. The half-lives of ^{134}Cs and ^{137}Cs are 2.1 and 30 years, respectively. Both these isotopes (and the daughter ^{137m}Ba radionuclide) emit beta and gamma radiations with peak energies of 0.6–1.4 MeV. The migration and availability of caesium radionuclides in the soil depend considerably on their physico-chemical composition. Caesium is transported most intensively by diffusion and convective diffusion processes within peat and sandy soils. These soils are also characterized by the most intensive transfer of caesium in vegetation. In contrast, in clay-rich soils microamounts of caesium are fixed strongly and are transported slowly along the biological chain. Considerably less ^{137}Cs is transported from dry land to water ecosystems compared to ^{90}Sr.

Both ^{134}Cs and ^{137}Cs emit penetrating gamma radiation, and are therefore potentially important contributors of external dose to humans. The dose rate of ^{137}Cs gamma

TABLE 3   Ingestion dose coefficients for different radionuclides and age groups (nSv of effective dose per Bq intake)

Radionuclide	Age (years)					
	< 1	1–2	2–7	7–12	12–17	> 17
^{90}Sr	230	72	47	60	79	28
^{134}Cs	26	16	13	14	19	19
^{137}Cs	21	12	10	10	13	14

Data from ICRP (1993).

radiation in the air decreases after radioactive contamination of dry land in moderate latitudes initially with a half-life of 1.5 years.

Like ^{90}Sr, the surface contamination of vegetation with caesium radionuclides decreases with a half-life of about two weeks. The transfer of ^{134}Cs and ^{137}Cs from soil to plants is generally only important several months after aerial contamination of the surface, when radionuclides are mixed with the soil. The caesium transfer factors from soil to vegetation can differ by up to two to three orders of magnitude, depending on the type and composition of the soil. Usually, the ^{137}Cs transfer factor decreases with a half-life of 1–10 years, and in 5–10 years this process slows down. About 1% of the ^{134}Cs and ^{137}Cs absorbed by a cow during a day is present in a litre of its milk. These isotopes are absorbed almost completely into the bloodstream of humans from the intestinal tract, and they accumulate, like potassium, within the cells of tissues such as muscles and parenchymal organs (liver, kidneys, etc.). Considerable quantities of caesium radionuclides concentrate in food products of forest origin (such as mushrooms, berries and game) and in fresh-water fish of lakes with a low mineral content. Table 3 presents dose factors for the incorporation of ^{134}Cs and ^{137}Cs in people of different ages (ICRP 1993).

Plutonium

Isotopes of plutonium, which have atomic numbers ranging from 238 to 241, have entered the environment as a result of the events shown in Table 1. ^{238}Pu, ^{239}Pu and ^{240}Pu are alpha emitters, with energies of radiation ranging from 5.1 to 5.6 MeV. Their half-lives range from 88 years to 24 000 years. ^{241}Pu emits soft beta radiation and has a half-life of 14.4 years, forming the alpha emitter ^{241}Am, which increases in the environment following a plutonium release.

Plutonium is a chemical analogue of the rare earth elements, and it is weakly soluble in natural conditions. If it enters the environment within radioactive particles it remains within the particles for many years, migrating through soil and water ecosystems by mechanical transport. Because of its low solubility in soil solutions, its transfer to plants and along the ecological chain to humans is insignificant. The main process of plutonium migration is wind resuspension and inhalation. In the immediate period after a contamination of dry land, the plutonium wind resuspension factor can be of the order of magnitude of $10^{-9}\,\mathrm{m}^{-1}$. It is assumed that the transfer of ^{241}Am from soil to vegetation is more intensive than that of plutonium isotopes.

Compounds of Pu and ^{241}Am inhaled by humans are retained in the lungs. Depending on their physico-chemical form, which can have a half-life ranging from several days to 1–3 years, they are dissolved in body liquids and transported to liver and bone tissue, where they remain for a long period of time. The inhalation dose coefficients for ^{238}Pu, ^{239}Pu, ^{240}Pu and ^{241}Am from the atmospheric air are about $1 \times 10^{-4}\,\mathrm{Sv/Bq}$.

Methods for monitoring internal exposure

Two different methodologies are used for the assessment of internal exposure dose in inhabitants of an area contaminated with radionuclides. In the first method, the dose is calculated from measurements of radionuclide intake from inhalation and from the consumption of water and food products. The data on content of radionuclides in soil, air, drinking water, agricultural and natural food products are obtained from current radiation monitoring and radioecological studies. The rate of inhalation by persons of different age, sex and profession is known from physiological investigations. The rate of consumption of different food products is dependent on age, sex, local traditions of agricultural production, gathering of natural food products and food habits. These data are usually obtained from population surveys and from analyses of statistical data. The dose factors are usually taken from the ICRP-67 report (ICRP 1993). This method also makes use of radiometric analyses of homogenized foods or daily excreta.

The second method involves measuring the radionuclide levels in humans. For the gamma-emitting nuclides ^{134}Cs and ^{137}Cs, whole-body counters (WBCs) have been the most widely used method since the 1960s. Stationary WBCs have been constructed in research centres of developed countries, and there are also portable facilities for on-site dose measurements. Calibration of the WBC is performed by means of anthropomorphic phantoms containing standard sources of gamma radiation. Internal contaminations with the beta emitter ^{90}Sr and the alpha emitters ^{238}Pu, ^{239}Pu, ^{240}Pu and ^{241}Am are determined by the analysis of autopsy samples of bone and other tissues. In Chelyabinsk a unique WBC has been operating for 20 years that is designed for measuring the ^{90}Sr/Y levels in people with bremsstrahlung. When the concentrations of radionuclides are low, they can be estimated from the excreta data using indirect dosimetry. All methods for measuring internal radionuclide levels require additional information on the dynamics of radionuclide intake for the calculation of the internal exposure dose.

The first method is more active and uses relatively simple equipment. Its drawbacks are that there are variations in the radionuclide content of air, water and foods, and that conservative average values of physiological constants have to be applied. Intakes and the corresponding internal doses are usually overestimated. The second method usually requires more complex equipment and it is not always active, as is the case for the analysis of autopsy samples. However, measurements of the radionuclide levels in people are more closely related to the internal exposure dose and they permit a more accurate assessment. The comparison of the two methods and the corresponding correction of dosimetric models is a subject of scientific interest.

Extensive information has been accumulated on the internal exposure of populations after major releases into the environment. The results of monitoring a number of contaminated areas were used to make decisions about radiation protection measures: for example, the prohibition of local food consumption and its replacement by radiation-free foods, changes in agricultural and food production, and resettlement of inhabitants to other areas.

Major releases of long-lived radionuclides into the environment and their effect on populations

The consequences of major radiation accidents described below demonstrate the importance of internal exposure from long-lived radionuclides.

Global fallouts

Table 2 shows that the bulk of ^{90}Sr, ^{137}Cs, ^{239}Pu and ^{240}Pu was released into the atmosphere as a result of nuclear tests. The radionuclides were gradually deposited on the earth's surface during the 1960s and 1970s. Twelve of the 22 radionuclides that made a significant contribution to the collective exposure of the earth's population due to nuclear tests have half-lives of over one year. All of these are sources of human internal exposure. The ecologically transportable radionuclides ^{14}C, ^{137}Cs, ^{90}Sr and ^{3}H were transferred to humans predominantly via the consumption of contaminated food, and the weakly soluble plutonium isotopes and ^{241}Am transferred via inhalation. Deposition of radionuclides transferred onto the surface of plants played an important role in the long-term contamination of vegetable and animal food products. There was a significant transfer of radionuclides from peat and sandy soils to plants via root systems, especially in Polesye, but an insignificant transfer from clay soils. In the majority of areas, ^{90}Sr and ^{137}Cs were transferred to humans mainly via the consumption of contaminated milk and cereals, although a significant proportion of ^{137}Cs transfer also occurred via the consumption of contaminated agricultural and wild meat. During the winter, an extraordinarily high concentration of ^{137}Cs was found in reindeer meat, which can be explained by its high interception and long retention by lichens.

The highest levels of ^{137}Cs in humans were found in the mid-1960s, and these subsequently decreased with a half-life of 2–5 years. The peak levels of ^{137}Cs in the body of adult inhabitants of the Northern hemisphere reached 0.2–2.0 kBq in temperate latitudes, 2–20 kBq in the regions of Polesye and 10–100 kBq in reindeer herdsmen of the Arctic. In this period the effective annual doses from incorporated ^{137}Cs in these three regions were about 0.007–0.070 mSv, 0.07–0.70 mSv and 0.4–4.0 mSv, respectively (UNSCEAR 1982, Marey et al 1980, Ramzaev et al 1993).

^{90}Sr incorporation in humans is less dependent on natural conditions than the incorporation of ^{137}Cs. However, its concentration in the skeleton does depend on age. In the temperate latitudes of the Northern hemisphere in the mid-1960s the annual effective dose in adults and children under 5 years of age was about 0.003 mSv and 0.01 mSv, respectively (UNSCEAR 1982, Marey et al 1980).

The per cent internal exposure to long-lived radionuclides contributing to the collective dose to the year 2200 has been estimated as 64%. ^{14}C accounts for 39% of the collective dose and the remaining 25% is attributed to other radionuclides, among which ^{137}Cs and ^{90}Sr are the most significant. The contributions of Pu isotopes and ^{141}Am to the collective dose are an order of magnitude lower than those of ^{137}Cs and ^{90}Sr (UNSCEAR 1993).

Releases of wastes into the river Techa (1949–1956)

The first USSR plant for plutonium production, Mayak (near Chelyabinsk), commenced operations in 1948. Its liquid radioactive wastes were released into the river Techa. In total, about 100 PBq were released, including 95 PBq in 1950–1951. Together, ^{90}Sr and ^{137}Cs accounted for 12% of this radioactive mixture, together with ^{95}Zr/Nb and ruthenium isotopes, for example (Table 2). The concentration of radionuclides in the Techa river in 1950–1951 reached 5 MBq/l. The populations of villages along the river (28 000 total inhabitants) were subjected to external exposure from water, water-meadows and irrigated kitchen gardens. Contaminated water was used by the populations for drinking, watering cattle and fishing, for example. Therefore, radionuclides were incorporated in the bodies of inhabitants via water, milk, fish and other local food products. Although a considerable proportion of population along the river Techa was evacuated in 1953–1960, inhabitants of its upper part received average doses to the whole body of over 1 Gy during 25 years, some individuals receiving over 2 Gy. Both the total dose level and the contribution of internal exposure to the dose level depend on the distance between the river head and a settlement. Thus, the average effective accumulated dose in inhabitants of the village Muslyumovo, located at a distance of 78 km from the river head, was close to 0.23 Sv, 30% of which was from ^{90}Sr. At distances of over 100 km the inhabitants received, on average, 0.03 Sv, 40% of which was from ^{90}Sr (Degteva et al 1994), 10% from ^{137}Cs and 3% from ^{89}Sr. Specific features of the exposure of inhabitants of the river Techa are the enhanced doses in red bone marrow and on bone surfaces, which exceed the whole-body dose by 1.5–15-fold. The dependence of ^{90}Sr in the skeleton (according to the WBC data [Kozheurov & Degteva 1994]) and in teeth on the year of birth of inhabitants of the village Muslyumovo reflects the increased retention of ^{90}Sr in the skeleton of teenagers and in teeth of children (Fig. 1). High dose levels received by the bone marrow caused < 100–900 cases of chronic radiation sickness in inhabitants

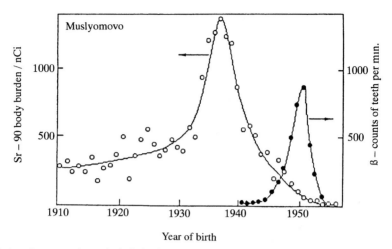

FIG. 1. Average values of whole-body counter measurements (○) and beta-count rates of teeth (●) for different age cohorts of residents of Muslyumovo (Kozheurov & Degteva 1994).

of the upper Techa in the 1950s and a higher incidence of leukaemia (UNSCEAR 1993, Degteva et al 1994, Kozheurov & Degteva 1994).

Marshall Islands (1954)

After the unexpectedly high power (15 Mt) thermonuclear test Bravo above the water near Bikini Atoll in the Pacific, several Marshall Islands were covered with a radioactive cloud. Like all fallouts of fresh products of nuclear fission, beta and gamma radiations of short-lived radionuclides was the main contributor to external exposure, and the intake of iodine radioisotopes that act on thyroid was the main contributor to internal exposure. This accident caused radiation sickness in the inhabitants of the islands and Japanese fishermen, and consequent development of thyroid tumours in children (UNSCEAR 1993). During the following years, the radiological problems were mainly concerned with the contamination of the islands with ^{137}Cs (Robinson et al 1994). The average levels of contamination in soil with ^{137}Cs, ^{20}Sr, ^{239}Pu/^{240}Pu and ^{241}Am were about 0.4 MBq/m^2, 1.5 MBq/m^2, 0.1 MBq/m^2 and 0.07 MBq/m^2, respectively. Exposure from ^{137}Cs contained in local food products was the main contributor to internal dose. A low level of exchangeable potassium in coral soil caused the intensive transfer of ^{137}Cs in coconuts and other food plants, and in pigs and hens. At the beginning of the 1980s, the average annual internal and external exposure doses from ^{137}Cs in inhabitants were about 3–4 mSv and 0.5 mSv, respectively. Over the next 30 years the expected external exposure from ^{137}Cs is 9 mSv, and the expected internal exposures (via the consumption of local foods such as coconuts) from ^{137}Cs, from ^{90}Sr, and from ^{239}Pu, ^{240}Pu and ^{241}Am collectively are

89 mSv, 1 mSv and 0.4 mSv, respectively. Measures to decrease the ^{137}Cs transfer to inhabitants are currently being developed (Robinson et al 1994).

The Kyshtim accident (1957)

The explosion of a tank with highly radioactive wastes at the Mayak plant in the Urals resulted in the release of about 70 PBq of a radioactive mixture in the air to a height of up to 1 km. ^{144}Ce/Pr and ^{95}Zr/Nb dominated the mixture, and long-lived ^{90}Sr contributed to 5.4% of the activity (Table 2). The radioactive trace with respect to the ^{90}Sr content on the soil mapped to a length of 300 km. The population (270 000 in number) was subjected to external exposure from gamma radiation caused by ^{95}Zr/Nb. Internal exposure of the intestinal tract was caused by ^{144}Ce/Pr, and of the red bone marrow and bone surfaces by ^{90}Sr/Y. Internal exposure resulted from the consumption of contaminated milk and local vegetables. Figure 2 shows the accumulation of the effective dose and of its main components in adult inhabitants, normalized to a ^{90}Sr soil contamination density of 1 Ci/km^2, according to the data of Nikipelov et al (1989). The contribution of ^{90}Sr/Y to the effective dose became more prominent 1–2 years after the decay of other radionuclides, and in 30 years reached 60% in the inhabitants remaining in the zone of the accident.

The 10 000 people who received the collective dose of 1300 person-sieverts were evacuated between seven and 670 days after the accident. The average effective dose in the most exposed group of evacuated inhabitants reached 0.5 Sv. Nevertheless, no negative medical consequences of the exposure to the health of the inhabitants residing in the zone of the Kyshtim accident were noted.

The Windscale accident (1957)

A month after the Kyshtim accident there was a fire at a reactor producing plutonium in Windscale, UK. During the three days of the fire, ^{131}I, ^{137}Cs and ^{106}Ru were released in the atmosphere (see Table 2), together with 8.8 TBq of ^{210}Po (UNSCEAR 1993). Residents of the UK and Europe were exposed mostly to ^{131}I. Internal exposure was limited by the early prohibition of the consumption of contaminated milk. Fifteen per cent of the total collective dose of 2000 person-sieverts was attributed to ^{137}Cs and 37% to ^{210}Po.

The Chernobyl accident (1986)

After nuclear tests in the atmosphere, the Chernobyl accident on 26 April 1986 was the most significant source of environmental radioactive contamination (Table 2). The explosion of a high power reactor and a consequent 10-day fire resulted in the radionuclide contamination of Eurasia, and especially the former USSR. The soil was contaminated with short-lived radionuclides, including ^{131}I, and the long-lived radionuclides ^{134}Cs and ^{137}Cs (and to lesser extent ^{90}Sr). Nearer the source,

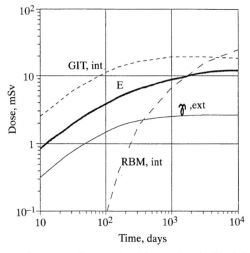

FIG. 2. Dose accumulation in adult rural residents after the Kyshtim accident in 1957. E, effective dose of internal (int) and external (ext) exposure; GIT, gastrointestinal tract; RBM, red bone marrow.

plutonium isotopes, and subsequently ^{241}Am, were the long-term sources of population exposure. Over 140 000 km^2 of the Ukraine, Belarus and Russia were contaminated with ^{137}Cs above 40 GBq/km^2, and over 7 000 km^2 above 600 GBq/km^2. The surface contamination of pasture vegetation caused the fast and high level contamination of local milk products with ^{131}I, ^{89}Sr, ^{90}Sr, ^{134}Cs and ^{137}Cs. Following the decay of short- and medium-lived radionuclides and the natural transfer of the surface contamination to the soil (i.e. from autumn 1986), the root transfer of ^{134}Cs and ^{137}Cs from the soil to vegetation and further along the food chain became the main route for the internal exposure of populations. From 1987 to 1991–1993 the transfer factors decreased in most contaminated regions, with a half-life of 1–2 years. The high level contamination of mushrooms and berries in forests of these regions did not decrease significantly over this period (Fig. 3). Therefore, natural food products have made a significant contribution to the internal exposure of populations over the last 3–5 years (UNSCEAR 1993, Merwin & Balonov 1993, Shutov et al 1996).

The quantities of ^{134}Cs and ^{137}Cs in the bodies of inhabitants in the contaminated areas reached their maximum levels in the summer of 1986. The average activities in some villages of the former USSR reached up to 0.4–0.6 MBq, and certain individuals may have been exposed to activities of up to 4 MBq. The average internal dose during the first year reached 5 mSv, and for certain individuals up to 50 mSv. A number of European countries had performed timely countermeasures, and in those regions the early incorporation was prevented. The peak activities in inhabitants of those countries were in the summer of 1987. The levels of ^{134}Cs and ^{137}Cs in the body decrease with a half-life of 0.3–2 years. Compared with the long-term external exposure, the internal

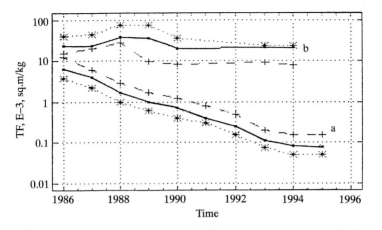

FIG. 3. ^{137}Cs transfer factor (TF) from soil to (a) milk and (b) mushrooms (*Boletus luteus*) in the Bryansk region as a function of time after the Chernobyl accident. Average values are given, and the 95% confidence limits are shown as dotted and dashed lines (Shutov et al 1997).

exposure dose is insignificant in black-earth regions, is nearly equal in turf–podzolic soils and is greater on peat soils in Polesye and in the Arctic. The contribution of ^{90}Sr, plutonium isotopes and ^{241}Am to the internal dose is insignificant. After the Chernobyl accident, large-scale agricultural and individual countermeasures were undertaken to protect the USSR populations from long-term internal exposure (UNSCEAR 1993, Merwin & Balonov 1993, Shutov et al 1996).

Tomsk-7 (1993)

In April 1993 the accident at the Siberian Chemical Plant resulted in the release of a mixture of fission products — including ^{95}Zr/Nb, ^{103}Ru, ^{106}Ru, ^{141}Ce, ^{144}Ce and ^{239}Pu — with a total activity of about 30 TBq (Table 2). A region of about 90 km^2 around the plant was contaminated, including a village with 73 inhabitants. The average dose during the first year in these inhabitants was 0.1–0.4 mSv. About 20% of the total dose was caused by inhalation. Due to the absence of ecologically transportable radionuclides in the mixture, no significant incorporation is expected in the future (Iljin et al 1995).

Discussion and conclusions

Table 4 presents an assessment of the collective effective doses in populations of the territories subjected to radioactive contamination in cases where internal exposure from long-lived radionuclides played an important role (UNSCEAR 1982, 1993, Degteva et al 1994, Nikipelov et al 1989, Iljin et al 1995). It also shows the per cent contributions in the total dose attributed to the incorporation of ^{131}I and the long-lived

TABLE 4 Collective effective dose following large radioactive releases into the environment (1000s person-sieverts)

Release	Area	Population ($\times 10^6$)	Total dose	Contribution of internal dose (%)	
				^{131}I in thyroid	Long-lived
River Techa, 1949–1956	Urals	0.03	10	ND	~40
Nuclear tests, 1952–1962	Worldwide	5×10^3	6700[a]	2	64
Kyshtim, 1957	Urals	0.27	3–5	ND	~50
Windscale, 1957	UK, Europe	ND	2	37	~5
Chernobyl, 1986	'Controlled'	0.27	20	25	25
	USSR, part of Europe	75	300	22	40
	Europe, Asia	ND	600	17	~35
Goiania, 1987	Brazil	0.001	0.06	ND	6

[a]Dose from ^{14}C estimated until the year 2200.
ND, not determined.

radionuclides ^{90}Sr, ^{134}Cs, ^{137}Cs, plutonium isotopes and ^{241}Am. For nuclear tests, we also took into account the contribution of ^{14}C until the year 2200, as in UNSCEAR (1993). The contribution of internal exposure from long-lived radionuclides to the collective dose and the corresponding population health risks as a result of major releases of radionuclides into the environment is significant (i.e. 5–64%). Disregarding the Windscale accident these values are 25%–64%. If thyroid exposures from ^{131}I are included the contribution of internal exposure reaches 40–66%.

The greatest collective dose from the incorporation of long-lived radionuclides was received as a result of the global fallouts, the Chernobyl accident, the events at the river Techa and the Kyshtim accident. At least for the river Techa releases, the incidence of chronic radiation sickness in inhabitants in the 1950s and of leukaemia can partially be explained by the incorporation of ^{90}Sr and ^{137}Cs.

Apart from these cohorts, Arctic reindeer breeders received the greatest individual doses of internal exposure from long-lived radionuclides (10–100 mSv throughout their lifetimes from global fallouts). The inhabitants of the most contaminated areas and of regions with peat soils after the Chernobyl accident received 10–50 mSv throughout their lifetimes. In temperate latitudes in remote terms consumption of natural products (such as mushrooms, berries, game and lake fish) that concentrate ^{137}Cs have made a significant contribution to the dose.

Major releases of long-lived radionuclides are in most cases consequences of accidents or the testing of new techniques, and they have a probabilistic nature. In combination with specific natural and climatic features they can cause different radiological consequences. Therefore, for the analysis of the consequences, consideration of specific features of the source and of local conditions are equally as important as the knowledge of the internal exposures to humans in the environment.

References

Degteva M, Kozheurov VP, Vorobiova MI 1994 General approach to dose reconstruction in the population exposed as a result of the release of radioactive wastes into the Techa river. Sci Total Environ 142:49–61

ICRP 1993 Age-dependent doses to members of the public from intake of radionuclides. 2. Ingestion dose coefficients. International Commission on Radiological Protection Publication 67. Pergamon, New York

Iljin L, Kochetkov P, Savkin M et al 1995 Incident at the Siberian Chemical Enterprises (Tomsk-7), 1993. International Atomic Energy Agency, Vienna

Kozheurov VP, Degteva M 1994 Dietary intake evaluation and dosimetric modeling for the Techa river residents based on *in vivo* measurements of ^{90}Sr in teeth and skeleton. Sci Total Environ 142:63–72

Marey AN, Barkhudarov RM, Knizhnikov VA et al 1980 Global fallouts of nuclear explosion products as a factor of human exposure [Russian]. Atomizdat, Moscow

Merwin SE, Balonov MI (eds) 1993 The Chernobyl papers. VI. Doses to the Soviet population and early health effects studies. Research Enterprises, Richland, WA

Nikipelov B, Romanov G, Buldakov L et al 1989 Radiation accident at South Ural in 1957. Atomnaja Energija 67:74–80

Ramzaev PV, Miretsky GI, Troitskaja MN, Doudarev AA 1993 Radioecological peculiarities around the Novaja Zemlja (USSR) atomic test range. Int J Radiat Hyg 1:1–14

Romanov GN, Spirin DA, Alexakin RM 1990 Radioactive substances in the environment. Priroda 5:53–57

Robinson WL, Bogen KT, Conrado CL 1994 A dose assessment for a US nuclear test site-Bikini Atoll. In: Assessing the radiological impact of past nuclear activities and events. International Atomic Energy Agency, Vienna, p 11–24

Shutov VN, Bruk GY, Basalaeva LM, Vasilevitskiy VA, Ivanova NP, Kaplun IS 1997 The role of mushrooms and berries in the formation of internal exposure doses to the population of Russia after the Chernobyl accident. Radiat Protect Dosim 67 4:55–64

UNSCEAR 1982 Ionizing radiation: sources and biological effects. United Nations Scientific Committee on the Effects of Atomic Radiation, United Nations, New York

UNSCEAR 1993 Sources and effects of ionizing radiation. United Nations Scientific Committee on the Effects of Atomic Radiation, United Nations, New York

DISCUSSION

Whicker: Why was there no radiocaesium released in the Kyshtim explosion?

Balonov: Because the tanks that exploded contained high activity liquid waste especially processed to remove radiocaesium.

Aarkrog: I have a short question concerning the nuclear tests. Does the figure you showed us include the French and the Chinese tests?

Balonov: The figures for the radionuclide release and collective dose are not much higher when those tests are included because the main tests contributing to the dose were those carried out in 1961 and 1962 by the USA and Soviet Union.

Paretzke: You have presented us with a review of human internal exposures mainly by long-lived radionuclides, an example of which occurred at the river Techa. However, another major effect of internal exposures in populations has been the effect of radioiodine on the thyroid. Could you comment on this?

Balonov: Yes, thyroid cancers and hypothyroidisms due to radiation exposures were detected after the Bravo thermonuclear test in the Pacific. Recently, an increased thyroid cancer morbidity in children has been revealed in areas of Belarus, Ukraine and Russia that have been contaminated with radionuclides from the Chernobyl nuclear power plant. The latent period appears to have been very short, of the order of 5–7 years. The large number of cases, about 1000 in 1996, and their appearance in contaminated areas have eliminated any doubts as to their origin. In the early period after the accident, the thyroid doses, and especially the collective doses for Belarus, were somewhat underestimated. Together with the unusually short latent period, this was the main reason why the high incidence rates of thyroid cancer in children reported in Belarus in 1992 were not believed by the international scientific community. However, subsequent international studies corroborated these results. Recent dose reconstruction studies in the three countries that suffered the most have been performed by Prof. Likhtarev (for the Ukraine), Dr Khrush (for Belarus) and our group (for Russia), and have estimated the collective ^{131}I thyroid doses as $1.1–1.5 \times 10^6$ person-sieverts. About half of this collective dose was received by children and teenagers. This collective dose is in reasonable agreement with the observed thyroid morbidity.

Whicker: I am puzzled by the observation that for thyroid cancer we would normally expect a latent period of about 15 years, but these cancers are appearing much earlier. Is there a known explanation for this?

Balonov: There is a partial explanation. This aspect of human radiobiology has not been carefully studied before because there were only a few cases of thyroid cancers in children caused by radiation. Therefore, these are relatively new data. For example, the latent period seems to depend on the dose level. In the most heavily contaminated areas of Belarus (the Gomel region) the cancers started appearing in 1990–1991. In other regions they have only been appearing since 1992, and in some of the lower contaminated areas they have only been appearing since 1995.

Cigna: You mentioned that the 1000 thyroid cancer cases came from controlled areas. What do you mean by this?

Balonov: Only about 20–30% came from the controlled area, which was an official area restricted with a level of 0.55 MBq/m^2 of ^{137}Cs on the soil surface and in which active countermeasures have been applied since 1986.

Roed: From which countries were the 1000 cases obtained?

Balonov: At least 500 cases were obtained from Belarus, 300 from the Ukraine and 100 from Russia.

Cigna: Why were the peak levels of ^{90}Sr in teeth and bone displaced?

Balonov: Because vertebrae develop actively during the teenage period and retain bone minerals for many decades. Teeth develop actively in early childhood and also retain calcium and strontium for many decades. Therefore, the two tissues actively accumulate ^{90}Sr during different developmental periods.

Goldman: The different latent periods for thyroid cancer are also related to the age. This was shown by Conard (1984) in the Marshall Islands. In children the latent period for thyroid cancer is short, perhaps between four to seven years. In addition, the higher the dose, the shorter the latent period. There is a minimum time between exposure and appearance, i.e. the latent period for induced cancers. Therefore, it may take several years for any cancer to become evident. The 1000 cases are probably just the beginning of the curve, which may end up being fourfold larger.

Paretzke: What is the evidence for your statement that the higher the dose the shorter the latent period?

Goldman: There have been hundreds of animal studies that have been confirmed with all kinds of dose rate and end-point variations (see Thompson & Mahaffey 1986).

Paretzke: One has to be careful because if many animals are exposed to high doses there will be a higher total incidence. Therefore, if one observes tumours that are above the background rate much earlier, this does not necessarily mean that the average tumour time distribution will also be earlier at higher doses.

Goldman: If the time-specific incidence rates in different test groups whose doses are different are compared, the time becomes shorter as the dose increases, at least to a certain minimum latency period.

Roed: Your model included the inhalation dose. In the early period did you take into account that the inhalation dose indoors is less than that outdoors?

Balonov: No. We did not use the dose for the early period because we didn't have many measurements from that period. Therefore, we dealt mainly with whole-body radioactivity.

Streffer: I agree that these new thyroid carcinoma data were obtained only after the Chernobyl accident, but on the other hand similar data following the bombing of Hiroshima and Nagasaki have also been described. Ron et al (1995) have reviewed all the published data, which agree with experiences from Chernobyl. I can give some additional absolute data on thyroid cancer in relation to the population of Belarus. Between 1986 and 1989 the incidence of thyroid carcinomas was 0.1–0.3 cases/100 000 children per year. However, between 1990 and 1994 this incidence increased to 1.2–3.5 cases/100 000 children per year. In the most heavily contaminated areas this increase was more dramatic. The rate increased from about 0.3 cases/100 000 children per year to 3.5–11.7 cases/100 000 children per year. There's no doubt that this is due to radioiodine exposure. This is the only effect that we've observed so far.

I also have a question concerning the high radioiodine doses. Did you say that the individual thyroid doses in the most heavily contaminated regions were as much as up to 1 Gy?

Balonov: They may even be 10–50-fold higher than that. 1 Gy represents an average dose in a particular age group.

Streffer: For how long did they receive this high dose?

Balonov: Two months.

Aarkrog: Do the diets of those at Hanford have a higher level of stable iodine than the diets in Russia?

Paretzke: I'm not so certain that stable iodine intake protects against thyroid problems because in a recent nationwide survey in the Marshall Islands we've found that thyroid problems are prevalent even though these islanders receive stable iodine via breathing air and consuming fish.

Streffer: The doses with respect to radioiodine are much higher in the Marshall Islands.

Paretzke: I was not referring to radiation effects due to weapons testing in the 1940s and 1950s. The present observation shows that abnormalities and even cancer are now prevalent in this population. This has little or nothing to do with the previous testing but is due to another, hitherto unknown, cause.

Streffer: This is a different point because a genetic predisposition may be present. The question is whether we can decrease the dose.

Paretkze: The smaller the daily stable iodine supply the larger the thyroid becomes. In Germany almost a million young (drafted) men aged about 18 years were analysed for their thyroid size, and a correlation was found between the thyroid size of these young people and the distance from the sea. Close to the sea the thyroids were smallest, and in Bavaria (i.e. the measurements that were furthest from the sea) they were the largest. This does not necessarily mean an increase in the dose per unit intake. The dose is given by the uptake-related energy absorbed divided by the organ mass. Therefore, if the mass is also increased, the ratio doesn't change appreciably. Consequently, even in an area where there is only a small stable dietary iodine supply (i.e. small compared to the World Health Organization's recommended 150 g per day) and a high uptake factor (in Bavaria it may be around 0.6, compared to the International Commission on Radiological Protection's recommended value of 0.2 to 0.3), the masses may be as large as twice the nominal 20 g, i.e. 40–50 g. If a high uptake is divided by a larger mass, then the difference of the dose coefficients in a normal and in an iodine-deficient area will be within less than a factor of two.

Streffer: I agree that these aspects are complex, but I also think that if there is an insufficient supply of iodine then the risk of uptake of radioactive iodine is higher.

Roed: You seem to understand how thyroid cancer progresses with time. Could you tell me what the total amount of thyroid cancers would be within the next 50 years apart from the 1000 cases you have reported?

Balonov: Both Marvin Goldman and myself have estimated this independently. Our estimate was between 3000–4000 and his was about 4000.

Goldman: I have a question about the incidence. Have you done enough analysis to determine the minimum doses that caused an excess of thyroid cancer in children?

Balonov: It's too early to determine this. It's probably a relatively small dose because some of these cases were in areas that were not highly contaminated.

Paretzke: In Belarus most cases occurred in children who had a dose to the thyroid of less than 0.1 Sv.

Balonov: The concept of the collective dose works in those cases.

Paretzke: It's also a large population of children. Therefore, if one divides the cases of cancer by the number of exposed children the dose response curve for effect per exposed child still increases with increasing dose.

Goldman: It's a similar dose to the minimum dose of external X-ray irradiation that causes thyroid cancer in children, i.e. 6 cGy.

Paretzke: That thyroid dose estimate is necessarily rather uncertain. These children were irradiated with X-rays for about 30 min. If a child is sitting under the X-ray apparatus for 30 min and moving around its thyroid will be shielded to very different degrees. Most of these epidemiological data are from the 1950s and I'm not sure whether anyone can still produce a good model for thyroid exposure assessment.

Roed: Is it true that in Belarus there is a high deficiency of iodine compared to other places in the former Soviet Union, which would consequently lead to higher doses?

Balonov: Yes, some regions of Belarus are known to be iodine-deficient regions, but the main reason for the elevated cancer incidence is that they received high doses from incorporated ^{131}I. Refugee children in St. Petersburg that escaped from this area just after the accident had received up to 50 Gy, but this was the maximum.

Voigt: But there are many cases in areas, such as the Grodno and Brest area in Belarus, where there was not a high level of radiocaesium contamination.

Paretzke: That is why accurate calculations of the transport of different radionuclides in the environment and in food-chains are important. We also have to determine the time dependency and rate and height of the release from the source, particularly for iodine. Most of the iodine stored in the reactor was released with and soon after the noble gases. Therefore, the time dependency of the source term might only hold true for elements such as caesium.

Streffer: How good are the estimates of radiation doses to the thyroid on an individual basis?

Balonov: We have searched our databases and found that there were about 300 000 individual ^{131}I thyroid measurements in total in Belarus, Russia and Ukraine. There is some degree of uncertainty in these cases because of the different techniques of measurement, but this is the best method for reconstructing the individual dose. If we do not find a particular person on a database, then we look at earlier measurements of ^{131}I in local food products, especially in milk, and arrange a meeting with his/her parents to ask them what their child consumed in May 1986. I cannot eliminate uncertainty at the moment, it's relatively large.

Streffer: Do you also have these data for children from Belarus?

Balonov: Not personally. A group of my colleagues in Moscow at the Institute of Biophysics are still working on this.

Paretzke: We only have data on the levels of iodine in the thyroid at a few weeks after the accident for 15 children. For the remaining 430 children, our best estimate of individual thyroid doses has an error margin of at least a factor of three.

Streffer: Therefore, we can only say something about the average numbers of cases and nothing about the risk of individual cases. I am worried about this problem because for the risk estimates from Japan we have individual estimates of the doses and we can say something about the individual risk. In Belarus we only know average doses of a group of people and there are cancers in this area. An error margin of a factor of three is better than a factor of 10. I would be interested to know something about individual doses because we are studying and treating children in Germany who have thyroid cancer.

Balonov: This can only be determined by a collaboration between the institutions responsible for this area.

Prisyazhniuk: The incidence of thyroid cancer of children in the most contaminated areas of the Ukraine was 14-fold larger than expected. This refers to a small area, in which there were 52 000 children under the age of 15 at the time of the accident.

References

Conard RA 1984 Late radiation effects in Marshall Islanders exposed to fallout 28 years ago. In: Boice JD, Fraumeni JF Jr (eds) Radiation carcinogenesis: epidemiology and biological significance. Raven, New York, p 57–71

Ron E, Lubin JH, Shore RE et al 1995 Thyroid cancer after exposure to external radiation: a pooled analysis of seven studies. Radiat Res 141:259–277

Thompson RC, Mahaffey JA 1986 Life-span radiation effects studies in animals: what can they tell us? United States Department of Energy, CONF-830951 (DE87000490), National Technical Information Service, US Department of Commerce, Springfield, VA

General discussion III

Voigt: Has anyone calculated the costs of medical psychological treatments compared with those of remediation in the 30 km exclusion zone?

Roed: I went to a conference in Novozybkov, Russia in August 1994 during which the psychological effects of the Chernobyl accident were discussed. The stress symptoms described by the people in those regions were dependent on the contamination levels, but they were also influenced by the general situation in the different regions at the time of the investigation.

Gadd: In my opinion, if there is a real problem, psychology will not solve it. Thinking about the problem will not remove radioactivity or any of its potential effects.

Renn: I will present more information on this topic in my chapter (Renn 1997, this volume), but I would like to give a quick response. One interesting aspect in terms of looking at psychosomatic effects is that many of these effects lead to somatic symptoms. We can observe clinical illness not associated with any exogenous causing agent. We've seen these effects in many countries. It is difficult, even for clinical psychologists, to treat these people. The patients have their own version of causation. The causal change begins for them with an accident, and anything that happens to that person afterwards is attributed to that specific event. If you claim that the initial event could not cause the subsequent series of clinical symptoms, the whole mental chain would break apart. The patient would then respond with defensive mechanisms that allow him or her to sustain the hypothesized causal connections. If someone has a strict belief system on causation, s/he will only select information that supports his or her own view. Any counter-information, as valid as it may be, will be discarded because of a subconscious information-filtering system. There have been some experiments in which people have been exposed to clear arguments that contradicted their own position. When asked to repeat these arguments, they twisted them in a way so that they allegedly supported their original viewpoint. This is called 'reduction of cognitive dissonance'. The ability to influence this mental process is rather low. It's important that we don't overestimate the ability of psychologists to convince people that their assumed causal chain is not substantiated. Psychologists can work on this task, but it is an illusion to believe that once we tell patients the symptoms are possibly psychosomatic they would stop believing in their hypothesis, let alone that their symptoms would disappear.

Goldman: Were any countermeasures initiated immediately after the Chernobyl accident to reduce iodine exposure, and if so what effect did they have?

Balonov: More than 60% of the population of Pripyat, which is close to the Chernobyl power plant, took stable iodine the day after. We could estimate the effect of these countermeasures in this area because we measured the ^{131}I activity in the thyroid of 200 refugees from these areas and asked them whether they had taken stable iodine. The difference was in the order of one magnitude compared with most of the people living in Pripyat.

Goldman: And what was the situation in other regions, such as in Belarus, for example?

Balonov: Many of the people in these regions received iodine, although in most cases this was taken rather late. I would say that it wasn't an effective countermeasure. Probably the most effective countermeasure was that arranged in the Russian area of Novozybkov by the local sanitary inspection service, which prohibited the consumption of local milk at the beginning of May. According to our estimations, this decreased the dose to the thyroid by a factor of two. This is one of the reasons why we have a low level of thyroid cancers in Russia in spite of a high level of contamination. In other regions this countermeasure was not introduced effectively.

Streffer: Do you really think that this is the main reason for the distribution pattern of thyroid cancers?

Balonov: It may not be the main reason but it is a significant reason. It wasn't carried out in Belarus because there were no radiation protection experts there. The situation in the Ukraine was a little better, but most of the experts were sent to Chernobyl.

Häkanson: It's sometimes scary to compare the costs and benefits of countermeasures. For example, the typical cost of potash treatments of a lake is about US$30 000 per lake (about 1 km^2), it would take about four years to complete and it would lower the caesium levels in predatory fish by a maximum of 5%. There may be other benefits of potash treatment, but if it is done purely for radioecological reasons it can be extremely expensive.

Reference

Renn O 1997 Mental health, stress and risk perception: insights from psychological research. In: Health impacts of large releases of radionuclides. Wiley, Chichester (Ciba Found Symp 203) p 205–231

Interactions with human nutrition and other indices of population health

Arrigo A. Cigna

Fraz. Tuffo, I-14023 Cocconato A T, Italy

Abstract. The consumption of food is an important pathway involved in the internal contamination of humans. The site-related critical foodstuffs can be grouped into three main categories: dairy products; aquatic animals, such as fish, molluscs and crustaceans; and other typical foods. The concentration factor plays a more important role than the amount of a certain food consumed. Semi-natural and natural ecosystems are of special interest in this context because they can provide critical pathways for radionuclide transfer to humans, and they can also act as temporary sinks or long-term sources for radionuclides deposited from the atmosphere. From the viewpoint of population health, another important role is played by the countermeasures. The reference values commonly adopted in radiation protection are conservative and they have been established for planning practices that could provide future sources of irradiation. After a large release of radionuclides, the evaluation of the problem must be as realistic as possible, otherwise the countermeasures will imply consequences worse than those produced by the accident itself (without any further intervention). This criterion was clearly stated by the International Commission on Radiological Protection but it was frequently neglected after the Chernobyl accident. The results of a survey on the number of induced abortions following this incident are reported. These suggest that moral and ethical problems are involved above and beyond any economical implications.

1997 Health impacts of large releases of radionuclides. Wiley, Chichester (Ciba Foundation Symposium 203) p 141–154

Following a large release of radionuclides, food consumption plays an important role in the pathway resulting in the internal contamination of exposed humans. The dietary habits of the area being considered must be studied in order to identify the site-related critical foodstuffs. Once all the parameters concerning such foodstuffs are known, it is possible to adopt a reliable model to describe quantitatively the behaviour of the radioactive contamination in its pathway from the first local environment to the individuals in the critical group. The effective dose delivered to them can then be assessed.

The health of the population can be affected by factors other than nutrition. In particular, the effects of countermeasures can augment the role of nutrition. Such effects can also be apparent outside the domain of radiation protection, as was found after the Chernobyl accident.

Foodstuff categories

The relevant foodstuffs can be grouped into three main categories: dairy products; aquatic animals, such as fish, molluscs and crustaceans; and other typical foods. The experience of many years of study confirms that the contribution due to some kinds of food, such as cereals, that are consumed frequently is not relevant because the concentration factor of the radionuclides is relatively small. In other words, the concentration factor plays a more important role than the amount of a certain food consumed. By taking into account this criterion, the identification of the critical foods for a certain population is simplified and, in general, does not require time-consuming research.

Dairy products are mostly derived from cows fed on a semi-industrial basis. Therefore, their contamination is largely determined by the evolution of the radionuclides deposited on agricultural environments. The processes that affect the transfer of radionuclides within the terrestrial biosphere can be conveniently described by compartment models. Obviously the time of the year when the contamination occurred, together with the agricultural practice, can influence the transfer of radionuclides. Therefore, as stated by the OECD-NEA (1989), the influence of seasonal conditions must be taken into account.

Generally, milk and dairy products from sheep and goats are more contaminated than those obtained from cows because sheep and goats feed on grass that is closer to the ground and more easily contaminated with soil particles. However, as a consequence of a faster metabolism, their internal contamination disappears in a relatively short period, i.e. of the order of some weeks after they stop feeding on contaminated grass.

Aquatic edible animals, as well as other typical foods (e.g. mushrooms and game) are more commonly found in semi-natural and natural ecosystems. Animals such as game and fish have a seasonal choice of food. In the case of some species of fresh-water fish, contamination of the high trophic levels may persist for a long time (years) if the water turnover is relatively slow. This may be caused by the geohydrological characteristics of the basin (e.g. absence of outlets) or the climatic conditions (e.g. presence of ice) (OECD-NEA 1991).

One foodstuff with a rather irregular contamination is honey. For most samples of honey obtained after the Chernobyl accident, the concentrations of ^{134}Cs and ^{137}Cs were relatively low because of the selective processes in the food-chain: flower→nectar→bee→ honey. However, there was a higher concentration of ^{134}Cs and ^{137}Cs in some samples, such as those obtained from bees collecting honeydew instead of nectar (Mercuri 1988). Honeydew is a sweet liquid left on plants by insects that suck lymph and it behaves as a trap for atmospheric particles.

Mushrooms, in general, are more contaminated than other foodstuffs. Some species (e.g. *Boletus badius, Boletus scaber* and *Boletus subtomentosus*) have a concentration of ^{134}Cs and ^{137}Cs higher (up to one order of magnitude) than other mushroom species of the same genus. This could be due to the development of their respective mycelia in layers at different depths, the ones closer to the surface being more easily contaminated by radioactive fallout.

It is evident that semi-natural ecosystems can provide critical pathways for radionuclide transfer to humans, and they can also act as temporary sinks or long-term sources for radionuclides deposited from the atmosphere. Further research and modelling is therefore necessary (Coughtrey et al 1991).

Countermeasures

From a population health viewpoint, another important role is played by countermeasures. The reference values commonly adopted in radiation protection are conservative and they have been established for planning practices that could provide sources of irradiation in the future. After a large radionuclide release, the evaluation of the problem must be as realistic as possible, otherwise the countermeasures will result in consequences worse than those produced by the accident itself without further intervention. Therefore, the two categories of situations need different handling at the regulatory level (Dunster 1987). This criterion was clearly stated by the International Commission on Radiological Protection (ICRP), but it was frequently neglected after the Chernobyl accident.

Under normal operational conditions, the individual dose limit for the public recommended by the ICRP (1990, 1991) is 1 mSv per year, but in special circumstances a higher value of effective dose could be allowed in a single year, provided that the average over five years does not exceed 1 mSv per year.

In serious accidents some relaxation of the controls for normal situations can be permitted without lowering the long-term level of protection. This is a consequence of two key concepts: (1) deterministic effects are not likely to occur at absorbed doses of less than 0.5 Gy; and (2) the benefit corresponding to the dose saved by implementing a protective action (averted dose) must be greater than the risk as a consequence of the protective action.

The intervention levels recommended by the ICRP (1993) are summarized in Table 1. After a severe accident, measures must be taken to minimize the consequences of the accident, taking into account the optimization principle. Certain interventions may have serious health or socioeconomic consequences to the individual or society; others have only little impact, although there are no interventions that are not associated with some disadvantages.

The estimations of the average individual effective dose caused by the Chernobyl accident for the first year in different countries have not exceeded 5 mSv (and in most cases these were lower by some orders of magnitude). The introduction of countermeasures below this level is not warranted by a virtually unanimous

TABLE 1   International Commission on Radiological Protection (1993) recommended intervention levels

Type of intervention	Intervention level of averted dose	
	Almost always justified (mSv)	Range of optimized values
Sheltering	50	Not more than 10-fold lower than the justified value
Administration of stable iodine: equivalent dose to thyroid	500	Not more than 10-fold lower than the justified value
Evacuation (<1 week): whole-body dose	500	Not more than 10-fold lower than the justified value
equivalent dose to skin	5000	Not more than 10-fold lower than the justified value
Relocation	1000	5–15 mSv per month for prolonged exposure
Restriction to a single foodstuff	10 (in one year)	1000–10 000 Bq/kg (beta/gamma emitters) and 10–100 Bq/kg (alpha emitters)

agreement among several international organizations (Cigna 1989). Countermeasures that have been endorsed in many countries are not justified because their cost was higher than the advantage obtained by the dose reduction. In the case of Chernobyl, only in the vicinity of the plant were the limits substantially exceeded, and only there did the countermeasures provide a net benefit for the population. More generally, as was stated clearly by the OECD-NEA (1987), protective actions that were often taken largely on the basis of non-radiological criteria rather than on true radiation protection requirements had a negative influence.

'Maximum permitted levels' for foodstuffs

As a historical case, the situation after the Chernobyl accident is a typical example of an aberrant behaviour of the authorities, who should have implemented the wise recommendations of the ICRP (which already existed, if not in their final version quoted above) with the support of the operational experience of radiation protection experts.

At first, the Commission of the European Communities issued a 'recommendation of the commission' (Table 2), which was quite unrealistic both in form (because a limit not related to specified radionuclides in a mixture of radionuclides with a wide range of half-lives and energies was meaningless) and in content (because too large a number of samples already exceeded the limits for the global amount of gamma emitters and therefore it was nonsense to forbid the consumption of foodstuffs in a large area

TABLE 2   Maximum permitted levels of radioactivity in foodstuffs which may be marketed

Date[a]	Maximum activity (Bq/kg)	
	Dairy produce	Fruit and vegetables
6 May 1986	500	350
16 May 1986	250	175
26 May 1986	125	90

[a]Date from which the limits reported in the table have to be observed.
Recommended by the Commission of the European Communities (Recommendation 86/156/CEE of 6 May 1986, published in the Official Journal of 7 May 1986).

without sound health reasons). In addition, the recommended levels were not consistent because dairy produce values, which should have been more conservative because dairy foods are the only food source for babies, were higher than those for fruits and vegetables.

Long discussions ensued, and it took some time before an agreement was reached among the member countries. The first regulation was issued at the end of May 1986 (Table 3). Unfortunately, these values were also determined for political reasons without a real scientific basis. In fact, in the following months the experts convened under Article 31 of the EURATOM Treaty proposed a new set of reference levels that were much more consistent from the point of view of radiation protection and were nearly 50-fold higher than the previous ones; however, the politics overruled the science.

It was assumed that the levels of intervention had to be chosen for the most sensitive part of the population, and for the more radiotoxic nuclides among each of four different groups of radionuclides. It was also assumed that each of the three different groups of foods were contaminated to the maximum extent. In the frame of the EURATOM Treaty, the Council took longer than two years to issue four regulations covering the different kinds of foodstuffs. In case of a nuclear accident, these maximum permissible levels will be applied for the shortest period possible and, in any case, for no longer than three months, unless a different recommendation is made by the Council itself. However, the levels established in May 1986 have not been replaced by the new ones, as everyone expected. The present situation is that they will be applied on 31 March 2000. The Council regulations adopted in the frame of the EURATOM Treaty will never be applied in practice because these levels (notwithstanding that they are exceedingly overprotective) are slightly higher that those established after the Chernobyl accident, and it would be rather difficult to explain this change to the public.

Concerning the rest of the world, the Codex Alimentarius Commission (a joint body of the World Health Organization, and Food and Agriculture Organization) adopted guideline levels (which are, in general, close to the EURATOM levels) for radioactive contamination of foods by assuming that the total amount of foodstuffs would be contaminated at the adopted values. However, radioactivity measurements in people after the Chernobyl accident and comparisons with food contamination confirmed the hypothesis that only a minor fraction of food was contaminated. The way in which intervention levels after the Chernobyl accident have been defined is an instructive example by itself of how one should not proceed.

The levels reported in Table 3 are intended for use in regulating the international trade of food. When these levels are exceeded, governments should decide whether, and under what circumstances, the food should be distributed within their jurisdiction. The proposed levels are intended to apply to artificial radioactive contamination of foodstuffs traded internationally and not to naturally occurring radionuclides that have always been present in the diet.

On the one hand, the Codex Alimentarius levels may imply an undue burden if the values are used overprotectively; but, on the other hand, the differences with respect to the Chernobyl and EURATOM levels show clearly that such values do not correspond to a clear line between 'safe' and 'unsafe', rather they only indicate a trend.

There is a basic difference between 'levels' and 'limits'. A level implies a lower and upper dose value for intervention that is dependent on the particular situation and is calculated in a realistic manner. In contrast, a limit is a boundary between exposures that are allowed and those that are not, and it is evaluated in a conservative manner. It is regrettable that in the directive from the Commission (and those of other agencies) only one value is given and this is, incorrectly, called the 'maximum level'. It should be defined as a level below which no action should be taken. However, this designation is a concession to the fact that this value has to serve to monitor food that will be marketed, exported or imported.

Health effects

It is difficult to convince the public that the first limits adopted by political and administrative authorities were too low and that the much higher limits, proposed by the experts, were defined in the very interest of the population without any other bias. Such a problem is difficult to solve because it cannot be dealt with on a purely logical basis. The risk perception by people does not correspond to facts, and an improvement of this risk perception cannot be foreseen in the future. The public, therefore, has to cope with an unjustified burden as a result of countermeasures, for example, in addition to the burden resulting directly from an accident itself.

Any action that is overprotective (i.e. that is not optimized by having a negative risk–benefit balance) implies, by definition, a cost that is not covered by any advantage. A dose reduction below values that are already negligible corresponds to a waste of money because no positive gain can be ensured. It must be remembered here that the consequences of excessive countermeasures may also result in severe harm and,

TABLE 3 Maximum permitted levels of radionuclides for foodstuffs and feeding-stuffs that may be marketed (excluding naturally occurring radionuclides)

| | | | | Maximum permitted level (Bq/kg) | | | |
| | | | | EURATOM | | | |
Foodstuff	Artificial radioisotopes	CEC[a]	WHO/FAO Codex AL[b]	3954/87[c]	944/89[d]	2218/89[e]	760/90[f]
Baby foods	Strontium			75			100
	Iodine			150			100
	Alpha emitters			1			1
	Caesium			400			1000
Dairy produce	Strontium		125				100
	Iodine		500				100
	Alpha emitters		20				1
	Caesium	370	1000				1000
Others (except for minor foodstuffs)	Strontium		750				100
	Iodine		2000				1000
	Alpha emitters		80				10
	Caesium	600	1250				1000
Minor foodstuffs	Strontium			7 500			
	Iodine			20 000			
	Alpha emitters			800			
	Caesium	600		12 500			
Liquid foodstuffs	Strontium				125		
	Iodine				500		
	Alpha emitters				20		
	Caesium	600			1000		
Feeding-stuffs:							
pigs	Caesium					1250	
poultry/ lambs/ calves	Caesium					2500	
others	Caesium					5000	

[a]CEC (Commissions of the European Community) 1707/86, 30 May 1986. The validity of these levels has been prolonged six times. They will be applied from 31 March 2000.
[b]WHO/FAO Codex AL (World Health Organization/Food and Agricultural Organization Codex Alimentarius Commission) 12 July 1989.
[c]22 December 1987.
[d]12 April 1989.
[e]18 July 1989.
[f]29 March 1990.

therefore, moral and ethical problems are involved above and beyond any economical implications.

The most widespread public health effects are probably psychological stress and anxiety, which may cause physical symptoms and affect health in a variety of ways (although such symptoms are unrelated to radiation exposure). This effect is a consequence of the public's perception of radioactivity as having fatal consequences at any level, and that they cannot protect themselves. It is difficult to educate the public to adopt a correct perspective in terms of radioactivity, but there are no other alternatives.

A survey of induced abortions in some European countries was carried out using the available literature to investigate the occurrence of more serious health implications. The frequency of induced abortions varies within a given year and within a given month of a particular year, suggesting that there are a number of confounding factors affecting the frequency of abortions. In addition, in some countries the statistical data concerning abortions differ according to the source, and therefore they are not reliable. In some cases it may be more useful to consider reliable birth rate data to estimate the increase of induced abortions. These data are summarized in Table 4.

In Hungary the percentage of induced abortions was not significantly higher in 1986 than in the preceding years. Nevertheless, a decrease of about 8000 births in the first three months of 1987 could be correlated with an equivalent increase of induced abortions in September 1986 and October 1986.

In Italy the decrease of about 3500 births in the first three months of 1987 (Cigna 1989) can be attributed to fewer planned conceptions, as well as to an increase of induced abortions in the previous year. This is in agreement with the results of Bertollini et al (1990) and Spinelli & Osborne (1991). Bertollini et al (1990) applied a linear regression model to the monthly birth data in 1977–1986 to calculate the expected births during the first three months of 1987, whereas Spinelli & Osborne (1991) used four regression models fitted to data of the monthly induced abortions between January 1984 and April 1986 to predict the expected number of abortions in the five months following the Chernobyl accident.

In Norway there was an increase of 192 spontaneous abortions in the year following May 1st 1986 with respect to the preceding year, and a decrease of planned conceptions during the three months after the accident. Both occurrences could be attributed to the stress caused by the situation.

In Sweden, according to Odlind & Ericson (1991), the increase reported for 1986 by Källén (1988) is not a consequence of the Chernobyl accident because the increase started before and continued far beyond the time of the accident. There was also an increase in the number of births a couple of years after the accident.Therefore, it seems unlikely that the fear of the consequence of radioactive fallout resulted in any substantial increase in the number of legal abortions in Sweden.

In conclusion, if in some countries induced abortions are not attributable to the concern expressed about the possible damage to the fetuses, then in other countries the politicians (ranging from local authorities up to government ministers) must be responsible for the public's confusion (which in some cases was closer to panic rather than to simple confusion).

If the detriment caused by undue countermeasures is taken either by ignorance (because they did not rely on the advice of qualified experts) or by demagogy

TABLE 4 **Abortions and births in some European countries after the Chernobyl accident**

Country	Increase in abortions		Increase in births	References
	Measured	Estimated		
Denmark	230	ND	ND	Knudsen 1991
Finland	0	ND	350	Harjulehto et al 1991
Greece	ND	2500	ND	Trichopoulos et al 1991
Hungary	0	?[a]	about 8000	Czeizel & Billege 1988 Czeizel 1991
Italy	ND	about 2000	about 3500	Cigna 1989
	ND	ND	5800	Bertollini et al 1990
	2600–8000	ND	ND	Spinelli & Osborne 1991
Norway	0		about 100	Irgens et al 1991 Egil Skjeldestad et al 1992
Sweden	500–600	ND	ND	Källén 1988

[a] The authors reported that they were unable to give an estimate.
ND, not determined.

(because they took decisions that accounted for themselves and not for the net benefit of the public), and if it is beyond any economical implication or results in severe health effects (such as the induced abortions reported before), the authorities must respond personally for their decision. Otherwise, the authorities will continue to be considered as being responsible for normal human error.

The termination of otherwise wanted pregnancies is a capital crime. Radiation protection experts are, therefore, for these moral and ethical reasons, obliged to oppose any wrong decisions.

Conclusion

It is easy to identify mistakes and incorrect procedures followed in many instances after the Chernobyl accident. The most appropriate ways to avoid such errors can then be identified. One problem, however, is that the public's reaction is often emotional and not logical. It is the view of many experts involved in the environmental measurements made after the Chernobyl accident that co-operation between competent and independent bodies from different countries would help to solve many of the problems and would establish effective guidelines in the event of future accidents.

The public authorities have held a large number of meetings concerning the problem of serious nuclear accidents with far-reaching implications, and they do have the tools for combined actions. They have also been informed that the reference levels issued by different bodies are over-protective and, therefore, that such values should not be considered as a sharp divide between what is 'safe' and 'unsafe'.

The ICRP recommendations (ICRP 1993) are adequate for planning the best protection of the public in a severe radiological emergency. These recommendations should be fully implemented. Any decision not strictly based upon radiation protection criteria should be avoided.

The lesson learned from the Chernobyl accident is that a major nuclear accident has only a few, if any, public health implications (that is, outside the local area). Therefore, a large amount of money could be wasted on over-protective actions. For these reasons, even though many hold the opposite view, nuclear accidents do not rank among the most threatening problems for humanity and the environment.

Acknowledgement

I thank Mercedes Catella for her invaluable help in providing many of the publications useful for this paper.

References

Bertollini R, Di Lallo D, Mastroiacovo P, Perucci CA 1990 Reduction of births in Italy after the Chernobyl accident. Scand J Work Environ Health 16:96–101

Cigna A 1989 Lesson learned and evaluation of the impact from the Chernobyl accident. In: Standing conference on health and safety in the nuclear age: second meeting: informing the public on improvements in emergency preparedness and nuclear accident management. Proceedings of a conference held in Brussels, 5 and 6 December 1989. Office for Official Publications of the European Communities, Luxembourg

Coughtrey PJ, Kirton JA, Mitchell NG 1991 Evaluation of food chain transfer data for use in accident consequences assessment. Proceedings of the seminar on methods and codes for assessing the off-site consequences of nuclear accidents, Athens 7–11 May 1990. Office for Official Publications of the European Communities, Luxembourg

Dunster HJ 1987 The place of optimisation in the setting of action levels for intervention following an accident. Proceedings of the International Scientists seminar on foodstuffs intervention levels following a nuclear accident, CEC, Luxembourg, 27–30 April 1987. Office for Official Publications of the European Communities, Luxembourg

ICRP 1990 Recommendations of the International Commission on Radiological Protection Publ. 60 Ann ICRP 21:46

ICRP 1991 Principles for intervention for protection of the public in a radiological emergency. International Commission on Radiological Protection Publ. 63 Ann ICRP 22:1–30

Källén B 1988 Pregnancy outcome in Sweden after Chernobyl: a study with central health registries. The Swedish National Board of Health, Stockholm

Mercuri AM 1988 Piogge polliniche nei mieli e inquinamento atmosferico: florula pollinica e presenza di cesio in un miele del 1986. Atti III Congresso Nazionale Associazione Italiana diAerobiologia, Pavia, 21–22 Sett 1988, p 273–275

Odlind V, Ericson A 1991 Incidence of legal abortion in Sweden after the Chernobyl accident. Biomed & Pharmacother 45:225–228

OECD-NEA 1987 The radiological impact of the Chernobyl accident in OECD countries. Organization for Economic Cooperation and Development, Paris

OECD-NEA 1989 The influence of seasonal conditions on the radiological consequences of a nuclear accident. Organization for Economic Cooperation and Development, Paris
OECD-NEA 1991 Influence of seasonal and meteorological factors on nuclear emergency planning. Organization for Economic Cooperation and Development, Paris
Spinelli A, Osborne JF 1991 The effects of the Chernobyl explosion on induced abortion in Italy. Biomed & Pharmacother 45:243–247

DISCUSSION

Voigt: I would like to make a small remark concerning honey. The relatively high activities in honey depend on the regions where the bees collect pollen. For example, in Germany we are still finding 50 Bq/kg in honey produced in forest areas 10 years after the accident.

Cigna: A high level is also found in honey produced from heather.

Konoplev: I would like to make a suggestion for further work in this area, i.e. that a comparison be made of the concentration in fish from different areas. For example, it would be interesting to compare the concentrations in fish from the northern part of the Kiev reservoir, which is inside the 30 km exclusion zone, with lakes in Europe. One might expect the concentration in fish in the Kiev reservoir to be much higher than in lakes that are more distant from Chernobyl. However, this is not the case. Two or three years after the accident we measured the concentration in fish from Kiev, and it was low because the self-purification of ^{137}Cs was high. In contrast, in some European lakes— for example, Devoke water in Cumbria, UK or Lake Vorsee in Baden Württemberg, Germany—the concentrations of ^{137}Cs are still higher than the European permissible levels (i.e. 600 Bq/kg). This is also much higher than the levels in the Kiev reservoir. It's an interesting point that only measuring the distance between an area and the site of the accident or even deposition is not enough. Therefore, decisions about countermeasures must take into account the environmental conditions.

Håkanson: I would like to stress this point with data from lakes. The data from the International Atomic Energy Agency (IAEA)'s VAMP (VAlidation of Model Predictions) programme come from many lakes in which there are large predatory fish such as perch and pike. We have about four to five orders of magnitude variations in caesium concentrations in predatory fish without any correction for differences in fallout. If we make a correction for fallout among the lakes, there is still three to four orders of magnitude variations. In this field we often talk about the load factor (i.e. fallout), lake sensitivity and effects (i.e. the caesium concentration in predatory fish). There are many important lake sensitivity factors, e.g. potassium concentration of lake water, that regulate the bio-uptake and potential effects. The load factor often has less influence on the caesium concentration in fish than the lake sensitivity factors.

Paretzke: I would like to challenge Arrigo Cigna's statement that cereals are not nutritionally important. After the Chernobyl accident, one-third of the cereal harvest in a European country had an activity level of caesium in cereals that was above the European limit for marketing. Also, if an accident like the Chernobyl accident occurred three months later most of the German harvest would have been above the same market value. Therefore, there can be tremendous effects on both economy and nutrition.

Cigna: Cereals are obviously nutritionally important; however, they are not the major foodstuff involved in the ingestion of radionuclides. On the other hand, politicians must understand that a contaminated harvest is, *de facto*, diluted with foreign crops that are not contaminated because in our society the food supply is obtained from many different sources.

Paretzke: This is illegal in the radiation protection laws of most western countries.

Cigna: But the final result is the same.

Goldman: Politically speaking, dilution is not the solution to pollution.

Howard: Is the point you're making that the limits are too low?

Cigna: Yes.

Paretzke: If a particular foodstuff is contaminated with 1000 Bq/kg and one consumed about 1 kg of it per day then one would receive a dose of 3–4 mSv per year alone from ingestion of this radionuclide. In addition, those who are more heavily affected are most likely living in the contaminated area and are therefore also exposed to some degree of external radiation. Their total dose may be about 5–7 mSv per year from an accident. This is not too low according to the International Commission on Radiological Protection (ICRP) and IAEA recommendations.

Cigna: I agree that a dose of 7 mSv/year is not too low. When the Food and Agricultural Organization (FAO) and World Health Organization (WHO) established their limits, they assumed that the total amount of food consumed by the population was contaminated at those limits, rather than only a proportion of the food, as was ascertained in practice.

Paretzke: A limit of 1000 Bq of radiocaesium per kg of food was derived from calculations assuming that only one tenth of the food is actually contaminated, it only takes into account a period of one to two years, and each food category out of the five categories can contribute singly to the 1 mSv. Therefore, the 1000 Bq/kg limit in food products for radiocaesium is not too low if we want to protect the public against an additional exposure of more than 1 mSv per year.

Aarkrog: What I like about the WHO figures is that they only operate with orders of magnitude. The wrong impression of certainty is given when limits such as 1250 Bq/kg and 380 Bq/kg are used.

Cigna: I agree that the Commissions of the European Community limits give a wrong impression of certainty. The problem with the FAO and WHO values is that they are not interpreted as orders of magnitude. Therefore, a food with a concentration exceeding the limit of 1 Bq/kg would be considered contaminated. Instead of giving a single value as a limit, upper and lower reference values should have been established, so as to give an idea that there is not a strict border between safe and unsafe but more of a grey zone in-between. The ICRP and the Nuclear Energy Agency adopted this wise criterion when they defined the upper and lower reference dose values for the adoption of countermeasures.

Aarkrog: Although we could comply with these limits within the EEC, we cannot be sure that our products will be accepted outside the EEC. There are countries in the Far East where the limits are close to zero.

Streffer: On the other hand, the limits that have been set are more or less safe enough in order to prevent health effects and there is very little food that we throw away. This is a sign of the radioprotection safety standards. We as scientists are responsible for these safety standards.

Cigna: Unfortunately, in other countries, such as in Italy, large amounts of foodstuffs were destroyed. In addition, my fear is that countermeasures often have a bad effect. The authorities in many European countries made irresponsible decisions. For example, the increase in induced abortions shows that the public was frightened by such decisions. The authorities did nothing to avoid the panic and to explain both to the public and to the people engaged in public health (such as doctors who are not necessarily experts in radiation protection) the health implications of the Chernobyl accident.

Streffer: They were not necessarily frightened by the authorities. In Germany they were frightened by those medical doctors telling them that no child should be born in 1986. Some reporters gave such talks, and they were ignorant of both the radiobiological and clinical data.

Frissel: The point about imposing limits is a difficult one, and I don't see a solution. As an analogy, in the Netherlands the speed limit is 100 km/h. If you drive at a speed of 108 km/h you don't get a fine, but if you drive at 109 km/h you do. A limit has to be put somewhere and, unless we develop a better system, we cannot give another recommendation.

Goldman: I'm sympathetic to what you're saying, but we have to convince the public that the limits we endorse have a margin of safety. I don't want to use the word threshold, but let's just say it's a margin. Taking the speed limits again as an analogy, I would like to see a system such that for a speed of 100–101 km/h a different fine is given than that for a speed of 200 km/h. That is, in terms of radioprotection, there is a gradation of severity. I agree that there's no simple substitute for having a set limit. However, the limits of food uptake are based on certain assumptions, and if the assumptions are overly conservative, i.e. that you assume 1 kg of honey is consumed per day, then this should be taken into account.

Roed: An accident has happened, and we have to improve the situation. I wonder whether all these limits that have been imposed do actually improve the situation because to my knowledge this is not certain. I would like to see some more cost–benefit calculations of these limits.

Renn: In my opinion, the issue of a standard setting is more complex. In terms of public perception, one has to take into account that it is difficult to distinguish between the collective dose, where a small dose is multiplied by a large population and thus produces inflated numbers of potential victims, and the individual dose which shows only marginal risk increases even after a severe nuclear accident. For example, the US Department of Energy (DOE) published a collective dose figure of 28 000 cancer cases that could be attributed to the Chernobyl accident for all of Europe outside the Chernobyl area. This was reported in all the newspapers. If you divide the additional cancer cases by the number of exposed people, you obtain an increase in individual risk of roughly 0.02%. The anti-nuclear campaigners stressed the DOE's admission of 28 000 additional cancer cases, whereas the pro-nuclear people have emphasized that an individual's risk has increased from 20% to 20.02%, which is obviously negligible. These two messages were conveyed to an attentive public, which was caught between two allegedly conflicting messages. They could not decide who was right or wrong. In such a case most people attribute credibility to the most pessimistic source. They believe it is better to be safe than sorry. Therefore, politicians who emphasized the safe views and requested more stringent standards received a lot of public support. This cautious behaviour is not irrational, but rather justifiable if you're not a radiological expert.

Also, there is a lot of evidence, specifically in the USA, that an over-reaction to public allegations of being exposed to a risk, even if such a reaction requires plenty of financial resources, is normally cost-effective for the company compared to a strategy of ignoring or playing down the allegations.

Cigna: The cost–benefit scenario should be applied more widely. In particular, the politicians, or rather the decision makers, should always be aware of the consequences of both employing a countermeasure or not employing it, so that they can make an informed decision, instead of acting on a purely emotional basis.

Biological effects of prenatal irradiation

Christian Streffer

Universitätsklinikum Essen, Institut für Medizinische Strahlenbiologie, Hufelandstrasse 55, D-45122 Essen, Germany

Abstract. After large releases of radionuclides, exposure of the embryo or fetus can take place by external irradiation or uptake of radionuclides. The embryo and fetus are radiosensitive throughout prenatal development. The quality and extent of radiation effects depend on the developmental stage. During the preimplantation period (one to 10 days postconception, p.c.), a radiation exposure of at least 0.2 Gy can cause the death of the embryo. Malformations are only observed in rare cases when genetic predispositions exist. Macroscopic, anatomical malformations are induced only after irradiation during the major organogenesis (two to eight weeks p.c.). A radiation dose of about 0.2 Gy is a doubling dose for the malformation risk, as extrapolated from experiments with rodents. The human embryo may be more radioresistant. During early fetogenesis (8–15 weeks p.c.) a high radiosensitivity exists for the development of the brain. Radiation doses of 1.0 Gy cause severe mental retardation in about 40% of the exposed fetuses. It must be taken into account that a radiation exposure during the fetal period can also induce cancer. It is generally assumed that the risk exists at about the same level as for children.

1997 Health impacts of large releases of radionuclides. Wiley, Chichester (Ciba Foundation Symposium 203) p 155–166

Radiobiological experiments and clinical experience have shown that the radiosensitivity of mammalian tissues and organs is correlated with cell proliferation and differentiation. This is one of the reasons why mammals are especially radiosensitive during prenatal development. Radiation exposure through radioactive substances can occur by external irradiation or by internal irradiation after the radionuclides have been incorporated. For external irradiation, the radiation dose can be estimated comparatively easily when the radiation exists of penetrating γ-rays. For internal irradiation with α-rays and β-rays, it is necessary to know the uptake and further biokinetic processes in the embryo or fetus.

Internal irradiation of organisms that develop *in utero* can occur when radionuclides are incorporated by the mother and are taken up by the embryo or fetus by crossing the placental barrier. This transplacental passage can occur for most radionuclides that are taken up in an ionic form. Active transport processes are also possible. Radioactive isotopes of caesium, which have been the main radiation source since the nuclear accident in Chernobyl, can migrate easily through the placenta and are taken up by the embryo and fetus. Therefore, the embryo or fetus may have the same, or even a higher, concentration of radionuclides than the mother. A similar situation can occur for radioiodine, i.e. that there is about twice as much radioiodine in the fetus than in the mother, as long as the thyroid is not active in the fetus. However, radioiodine can be taken up by the developing thyroid in late fetal development to a much higher concentration (about 10-fold) than in the thyroid of the mother. Therefore, fetal radiation exposure is dependent on fetal development in general and, in some cases, on the development of specific organs.

It is necessary to discuss the following effects after a prenatal irradiation event (Strahlenschutzkommission 1984, UNSCEAR 1986, Streffer 1995):

(1)   death of the embryo or fetus;
(2)   induction of malformations;
(3)   induction of growth retardation;
(4)   induction of functional disturbances; and
(5)   induction of cancer.

The occurrence of these effects, with respect to their quality (i.e. death, skeletal malformation, brain dysfunction, etc.) and quantitative extent depends on the developmental stages at which the radiation exposure takes place. Therefore, it is important to discuss the following three important developmental periods.

The preimplantation period

In humans this lasts until about day 10 postconception (p.c.). Rapid cell proliferation takes place during this period. In addition, cells differentiate to form the trophoblast, which is necessary for uterus implantation and the development of the placenta, and the inner cell mass, from which the embryo and fetus will develop.

The major organogenesis

This lasts for almost up to the end of the second month p.c. in humans. The various organs and tissues are formed during this developmental period. At the end of organogenesis, an organism can be distinguished that has the morphological structures of a human.

The fetal period

This lasts for the remainder of the pregnancy. During this period many differentiation and growth processes take place in all organs and tissues. The development of the CNS and brain occurs during the whole prenatal developmental period, but cell proliferation for the formation of the cortex is observed during early fetogenesis.

The actual time periods differ in other mammals (e.g. mice develop within around 20 days) but the developmental processes and stages are similar. Therefore, radiation effects observed in mice or rats can be extrapolated to humans when analogous developmental stages are compared.

Death of the embryo or fetus after radiation exposure

It is generally assumed that irradiation during the preimplantation period can cause only the death of the embryo or fetus. Changes in cell proliferation of preimplantation mice embryos have been observed after radiation doses of at least 0.25 Gy (X-rays and γ-rays). An increased occurrence of degenerative processes is observed with increasing dose. These degenerative processes cause the death of the embryos if no recovery takes place after low radiation doses. Until a few years ago, no significant increases in the prevalence of malformations had been observed after irradiation during this developmental period. Therefore, an all-or-nothing process had been formulated, i.e. that embryos are either able to recover from the radiation damage completely and develop normally or they die. This suggestion was based on the pluripotency of the blastomeres during this developmental stage, i.e. single cells of the preimplantation embryo die and are replaced by neighbouring cells (Hall 1993).

More recently, it has been observed that malformations can also be caused by irradiation during these developmental processes (Pampfer & Streffer 1988). This has been observed in strains of mice that have a genetic predisposition. These results will be discussed later. Data about the radiosensitivity of these early embryonic stages have not been obtained in humans because the pregnancy is usually not known during this early developmental stage, so that if radiation damage has occurred the embryo is released by processes that resemble normal physiological processes.

A greater radiation dose is required during the later developmental stages to cause the death of the embryo or fetus, i.e. radiosensitivity generally decreases, with respect to lethal events, during development.

Induction of malformations after irradiation

A radiation exposure during major organogenesis can lead to malformations (Brent 1980, Strahlenschutzkommission 1984, UNSCEAR 1986). Many experiments with mice, rats and dogs have shown that radiation doses in the range of 100 mGy (ionizing radiation of low LET [linear energy transfer], such as X-rays or γ-rays) and higher radiation doses can cause teratogenic effects. The developing skeleton and CNS are especially radiosensitive (Strahlenschutzkommission 1984, UNSCEAR 1993), and microcephalies, exencephalies and hydrocephalies in mice and rats have been observed at doses of 200 mGy and higher.

Studies of the survivors of the atomic bomb explosions in Hiroshima and Nagasaki have shown that radiation doses of at least 0.3–0.5 Gy induced an increased rate of microcephalies in children who had been irradiated during the major organogenesis (Blot & Miller 1973). Teratogenic effects in humans have usually been observed after higher radiation doses than in rodents. Ocular developmental defects have also been observed in children who were irradiated as a result of these atomic bombings when they were undergoing major organogenesis.

Changes as a result of radiation exposure also occur in the skeletal system; for example, in the extremities, spine and ribs. Each organ system is most radiosensitive during the period when differentiation of the organs begins. This is valid for rodents, but it has also been demonstrated in human clinical cases (Strahlenschutzkommission 1984).

Macroscopic teratogenic effects cannot be induced after termination of the major organogenesis. Therefore, the scheme shown in Fig. 1 has been developed in order to describe the phenomena mentioned above (Fritz-Niggli 1991, Hall 1993). When a radiation dose is given in a fractionated or chronic modality during organogensis, the radiation effects are lower than after acute radiation exposures, when the same total radiation doses are compared (Konermann 1976, 1977, 1987).

Growth retardation after irradiation

Growth retardation can be observed in newborns after prenatal irradiation. Growth retardation of mice and rats has been observed after irradiation during any period of prenatal development. However, the most prominent growth retardation occurs after irradiation during the major organogenesis. This growth retardation can be maintained throughout the rest of the organism's life. In children the growth retardation of the brain and skull is pronounced after prenatal radiation doses in the order of 0.5 Gy. Pronounced changes of the structure of neurons in the brain of mice have also been found after X-ray exposure (Konermann 1987).

The high radiosensitivity of the CNS can be explained by both the long developmental period of the brain and its complexity. Further, it appears that the CNS has more of a compensation deficiency than other tissues. Reduced head circumferences have been observed following 0.2 Gy exposures in Hiroshima and 1.4 Gy exposures in Nagasaki (Strahlenschutzkommission 1984). Disturbances of organs that have long periods for functional maturation can occur frequently. This has been found in the brain and also in the liver and the gonads.

Comparisons of total doses received by either fractionated irradiation or acute single radiation indicate that fractionated irradiation has a lower effect on growth retardation and maturation disturbances of the murine neonatal brain. This growth retardation, achieved with daily radiation doses of 0.6 Gy (five fractions during the early organogenesis), was compensated by cell proliferation until the third week after birth. However, such compensation took place to a lesser degree when the irradiation was performed during the early fetal period.

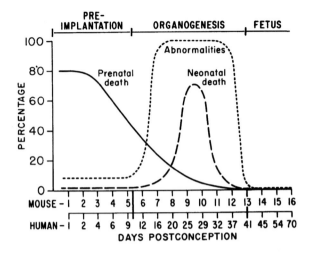

FIG.1. Schematic representation of the effect of radiation exposure at various developmental stages of humans and mice (data from Fritz-Niggli 1991, Hall 1993).

Functional disturbances after irradiation

The development of the CNS plays the most important role in this category of radiation effects. In rodents ionizing radiation induces disturbances mainly after exposures during the major organogenesis. However, the most radiosensitive phase of human brain development is during the early fetal period (third and fourth month of pregnancy) (UNSCEAR 1993). Clinical experiences after irradiation for tumour therapy, which have been performed during pregnancy, also show severe mental retardation in single cases. The most pronounced and impressive effects of this kind have been observed after the atomic bombings of Hiroshima and Nagasaki.

Severe mental retardation has been observed in 30 out of the 1544 children for whom prenatal radiation doses could be estimated. The highest risk existed for those children who were irradiated during the eighth to the 15th week of their prenatal development. A period of lower radiosensitivity existed during the 16th to 25th week p.c. An increased risk of severe mental retardation was not apparent in those irradiated before the eighth week and after the 25th week. The period of highest radiosensitivity coincides with the period of highest cell proliferation for the formation of the cortical neurons and the migration of neuronal cells from the location of proliferation to the cerebral cortex. Studies on the intelligence of children who were irradiated during prenatal development in Hiroshima and Nagasaki showed analogous results (UNSCEAR 1993).

Forty per cent of children who received doses of 1.00 Gy developed severe mental retardation. It is of special interest to determine if the dose–response curve has a

TABLE 1   Severe mental retardation of children after atomic bombing irradiation of
Hiroshima and Nagasaki at 8–15 weeks postconception (UNSCEAR 1993)

Radiation dose (Gy)	Number of persons	Number of cases	Per cent	Number of cases with Down's syndrome	Remaining per cent
<0.01	255	2	0.8	0	0.8
0.01–0.09	44	2	4.5	0	4.5
0.10–0.49	58	2	3.4	1	1.7
0.50–0.99	16	4	25.0	1	18.8
>1.00	12	9	75.0	0	75.0

threshold dose. This question has only recently been answered. When all children with
a severe mental retardation are included in the analysis of the dose–response curve, a
threshold dose of 0.40 Gy is obtained (confidence interval of 0.00–0.56 Gy). The lower
value of the 95% confidence limit allows a dose–response curve without a threshold.
However, three of the children with severe mental retardation were characterized as
having Down's syndrome, sufferers of which have a trisomy of chromosome 21 that
causes mental retardation. Two of these children with Down's syndrome were
irradiated during the eighth to 15th weeks p.c. The prenatal doses for these two
children were 0.29 and 0.56 Gy, respectively (Table 1) (Otake et al 1987).

The trisomies in the two children were not caused by irradiation because the
radiation exposure took place several weeks after the conception, when the genetic
defect was already manifest. Therefore, it is reasonable not to include these two
children in the analysis of the dose–response curve for severe mental retardation.
Under these conditions, a threshold dose of 0.46 Gy is obtained (95% confidence
interval of 0.23–0.61 Gy). With these data a dose–response curve without a threshold
dose can be excluded. In addition, considerations of the biological mechanisms that
lead to the mental retardation suggest that a dose–response curve without a
threshold dose is reasonable. On the basis of these data a dose–response curve with a
threshold dose in the range of 0.2–0.4 Gy for risk estimation is acceptable, although
further data are desirable for verification. It would have been reasonable had mental
development been analysed more carefully after the Chernobyl accident. It must be
stated again that the development of the human brain is sensitive at this stage and
therefore these effects deserve much attention.

Induction of cancer after irradiation

An association between childhood cancer and diagnostic X-rays during prenatal
development was described in the Oxford Survey Study of Childhood Cancers,
which was a large epidemiological study (Stewart & Kneale 1970). In most cases
diagnostic pelvimetric X-rays had been performed. In this study a relative risk for

TABLE 2   Mortality due to cancer in children exposed to prenatal diagnostic X-rays (Mole 1974)

| | Mortality (per 100 000 children) | | |
| | Single births | Twins | |
		Dizygotes	Monozygotes
Non-exposed			
Cancer	27	21	11
Leukaemia	23	16	0
Exposed to X-rays			
Cancer	39	31	29
Leukaemia	35	25	29

cancer during the first 14 years of about 1.4 was described for children who received an X-ray exposure during fetogenesis. However, other similar studies with a smaller number of cases produced different results. It was therefore assumed that the positive association between childhood cancer and diagnostic X-rays was due to a higher rate of complications, and this led to a selection bias. This bias was, however, excluded by comparing the association between childhood cancer and diagnostic X-rays in single births and twins (Mole 1974). Although the number of those who had been exposed to diagnostic X-rays was much higher in twins than in single births, the cancer induction rates were about the same in both groups (Table 2).

During the first years after the atomic bombing no increase in cancer was observed in those children who received an exposure to ionizing radiation during prenatal development. However, such an increase was found in a later study (UNSCEAR 1993, Yoshimoto et al 1988). In general, it is now accepted that the radiation-induced risk for the induction of cancer during prenatal development is within the same range as for exposures during childhood. This represents a two- to threefold higher risk than for adults (UNSCEAR 1993).

Genetic predisposition and induction of malformations

On the basis of the high recovery capacity of the embryo during the preimplantation period, it had been assumed that no malformations could be induced by ionizing radiation during this developmental stage. However, it has more recently been demonstrated that such malformations could be induced in mouse strains with a high genetic predisposition to these malformations by an exposure to ionizing radiation or alkylating agents (Generoso et al 1987, Pampfer & Streffer 1988, Müller & Streffer 1990).

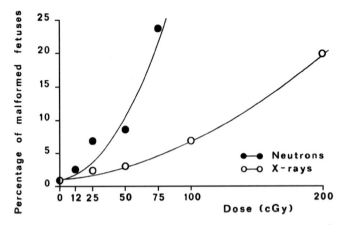

FIG. 2.   Induction of malformations (gastroschisis) after exposure of pregnant female mice to X-rays or fast neutrons at one hour postconception (Pampfer & Streffer 1988).

In a mouse strain that has a comparatively high spontaneous rate of the malformation gastroschisis, the Heiligenberger mouse, a radiation-induced increase in gastroschisis could be seen after exposure to X-rays and neutrons in a dose range of 0.12–2.00 Gy. Irradiation early after conception led to a dose–response curve without a threshold (Fig. 2) (Pampfer & Streffer 1988, Müller & Streffer 1990). Cross-breeding with another mouse strain and gene expression studies have shown that this effect is due to a genetic predisposition in the radiosensitive mouse strain. The relative intensities of a particular phosphocytokeratin were decreased in the liver, kidney and skin of those fetuses who developed gastroschisis after they had been X-irradiated one hour after conception (Table 3), suggesting that a genetic mechanism is involved (Hillebrandt & Streffer 1994). Two or three genes may be responsible for this effect (H. Hillebrandt & C. Streffer, unpublished results 1996).

TABLE 3   Relative intensities of a phosphocytokeratin in different organs in control fetuses and fetuses with gastroschisis 19 days postconception (Hillebrandt & Streffer 1994)

	Relative intensity [a]	
Organ	*Control* [b]	*Gastroschisis* [c]
Liver	10.11 ± 1.85	3.23, 3.45, 3.64, 3.75
Kidney	2.82 ± 0.40	1.76, 1.82, 1.96, 2.00
Skin	5.59 ± 0.63	4.08, 4.19, 4.23, 4.28

[a]Intensity of the phosphocytokeratin relative to the intensity of reference proteins.
[b]Mean of $n = 10$ fetuses of the Heiligenberger mouse strain $\pm$ S.D.
[c]Fetuses of the Heiligenberger mouse strain X-irradiated one hour postconception with 1 Gy.

These data demonstrate that the radiation damage is not randomly distributed in the genome of mammalian cells but that certain sensitive sites exist which are damaged more frequently than others after a radiation exposure. Therefore, certain weak points or 'hot spots' exist within the mammalian genome and radiation damage is expressed through radiation-induced alterations in these weak points.

In addition, the radiosensitivities of both humans and certain mouse strains exhibit a high degree of individual variability. This variability in radiosensitivity has been observed for a number of radiation effects in clinical experience and through cellular studies in the laboratory. It raises the problem of how to propose radioprotective regulations for those individuals who are highly radiosensitive. A number of ethical problems are included in such decisions which will have to be discussed in the future. Radioprotective regulations are presently orientated on the average radiosensitivity of large populations and not on the basis of individual variability.

Acknowledgements

These studies were supported by the Bundesministerium für Umwelt, Naturschutz and Reaktorsicherheit, by the European Community and by the Deutsche Forschungsgemeinschaft.

References

Blot W-J, Miller RW 1973 Mental retardation following *in utero* exposure to the atomic bombs of Hiroshima and Nagasaki. Radiology 106:617–620

Brent RL 1980 Radiation teratogenesis. Teratology 21:281–298

Fritz-Niggli H 1991 Strahlengefährdung/Strahlenschutz. 3. Auflage. Verlag Hans Huber, Bern

Generoso WN, Rutlegde JC, Cain KT, Hughes LA, Braden PW 1987 Exposure of female mice to ethylene oxide within hours after mating leads to fetal malformations and death. Mutat Res 176:269–274

Hall EJ 1993 Radiobiology for the radiologist. 4. Auflage. Lippincott, Philadelphia, PA

Hillebrandt S, Streffer C 1994 Protein patterns in tissues of fetuses with radiation-induced gastroschisis. Mutat Res 308:11–22

Konermann G 1976 Periodische Kompensationsreaktionen im Verlauf des postnatalen Wachstums von der Leber der Maus nach fraktionierter Röntgenbestrahlung während der Embryogenese. Strahlentherapie 152:550–576

Konermann G 1977 Periodische Kompensationsreaktionen im Verlaufe des postnalten Wachstums von dem Gehirn der Maus nach fraktionierter Röntgenbestrahlung während der Embryogenese. Strahlentherapie 153:399–414

Konermann G 1987 Postimplantation defects in development following ionizing radiation. In: Lett JT (ed) Advances in radiation biology. Academic Press, New York, p 91–167

Mole RH 1974 Antenatal irradiation and childhood cancer: Causation or coincidence? Br J Cancer 30:199–208

Müller W-U, Streffer C 1990 Lethal and teratogenic effects after exposure to X-rays at various times of early murine gestation. Teratology 42:643–650

Otake M, Yoshimaru H, Schull WJ 1987 Severe mental retardation among the prenatally exposed survivors of the atomic bombing of Hiroshima and Nagasaki. A comparison of T65DR and DS86 dosimetry systems. Radiation Effects Research Foundation, Hiroshima TR-1987

Pampfer S, Streffer C 1988 Prenatal death and malformations after irradiation of mouse zygotes with neutrons or X-rays. Teratology 37:599–607

Stewart A, Kneale GW 1970 Radiation dose effects in relation to obstetric X-rays and childhood cancer. Lancet 7658:1185–1188

Strahlenschutzkommission 1984 Wirkungen nach pränataler Bestrahlung. Veröffentlichungen der Strahlenschutzkommission, Band 2, Fischer-Verlag, Stuttgart

Streffer C 1995 Strahleneffekte nach Exposition während der pränatalen Entwicklung, Radiologue 35:141–147

UNSCEAR 1986 Genetic and somatic effects of ionizing radiation. United Nations Scientific Committee on the Effects of Atomic Radiation, United Nations, New York

UNSCEAR 1993 Sources and effects of ionizing radiation. United Nations Scientific Committee on the Effects of Atomic Radiation, United Nations, New York

Yoshimoto Y, Kato H, Schull WJ 1988 Risk of cancer among children exposed *in utero* to the bomb radiation. Lancet II:665–669

DISCUSSION

Prisyazhniuk: Is genetic predisposition involved in the manifestation of the effects of irradiation?

Streffer: This is not generally true, but the problem is that predisposition involves many recessive genes, so that if close relatives have children the probability that these recessive genes are inherited together is much higher. Therefore, the probability of a genetic predisposition to radiation sensitivity can be higher under such circumstances.

Aarkrog: Stewart & Kneale (1970) were also interested in these problems. Could you comment on their statements and compare them with your recent observations?

Streffer: I presented some of Alice Stewart's data on the Oxford Survey. Some of the analysis of these data was done by Mole (1974). There's no doubt that there was a radiation effect. However, Alice Stewart over-interpreted some of the data. She found eight cases with cancer after irradiation during embryogenesis, and she concluded that the effects were highest after irradiation during the first trimester of prenatal development. We have no additional data to support this statement. Further studies come from rodents and not from humans, and they do not show this effect. Mole analysed the data of single births and of twins. He argued that diagnostic X-rays were carried out only when there were complications, and that the leukaemia might therefore not have been caused by irradiation. As a result, Mole analysed single births and twins and he showed that the increase of cancer was more or less the same in both cases. However, only about 10% of the single births were exposed to diagnostic X-rays, whereas for twins there were more than 50%. Therefore, such a bias did not occur.

Paretzke: How do these numbers compare with the observations of leukaemia risks of those exposed *in utero* in Nagasaki or Hiroshima?

Streffer: This is another problem. For a long time, increases in cancer incidence were not observed in Nagasaki or Hiroshima. Yoshimoto et al (1988) showed that there was an increase, but this report was based on only a few cases. There is also a more recent publication which suggests that there was no increase (UNSCEAR 1993). Therefore, this matter has not been solved.

Paretzke: If we take the risk factors proposed by Alice Stewart we would expect in Hiroshima and Nagasaki to have at least 16 childhood leukaemia cases among the 1500 or so exposed *in utero*, but only one case was found.

Streffer: But the Oxford Survey is by far the largest population for which we have data available. There are 150 000 children, but in Japan there are no more than 1630 children. There are some cases but they are not significantly higher after radiation exposure than in the control group.

Goldman: One of the other important aspects of that analysis was that, although there were only a few cases involved, there was a crude linear dose–response relationship, i.e. the more X-rays taken, the greater the risk.

Voigt: Is there a test available to measure radiosensitivity that is easy to use?

Streffer: Unfortunately not. We are interested in developing such tests, but we must bear in mind that the reasons for the variability in individual radiosensitivity are complex. For instance, some cases may have a DNA repair deficiency and we may only be able to test the efficiency of one repair system. There may also be variations in DNA conformation, so that specific conformations have a higher radiosensitivity than others. It was believed for a long time that radiation damage was randomly distributed in the genome. However, more recent results have shown that this is not the case, and that there are certain weak points in the DNA which are more radiosensitive.

Renn: Did you see any evidence that, in addition to variations in radiosensitivity due to genetic defects, different individuals have different thresholds of sensitivity? For example, a threshold effect may be present in an individual whose DNA repair systems work well, but not in an individual who is characterized by deficient DNA repair symptoms. This threshold effect may vary depending on genetic predispositions of each individual.

Streffer: The understanding that we have so far is that this is unlikely. If there is a dose–response curve with a threshold, the curve can shift, and therefore the threshold can also shift. However, the presence of a threshold depends on the principle mechanism by which radiation effects develop.

Goldman: But in certain known genetic conditions, e.g. xeroderma pigmentosum, there are defects in repair such that a small dose of ultraviolet irradiation is efficient at inducing cancer (Cleaver 1968). It is a dramatic effect. It has been postulated that similar mechanisms may explain other ionizing radiation sensitivities.

I would like to raise another point. It is known that certain radionuclides, when present in the mother's blood, are transferred poorly across the placenta. For example, the mother can have between four- and 10-fold as much radiostrontium in her blood as the fetus, whereas for radioiodine and radiocaesium the concentrations are about equal. For other radionuclides, such as tritium, the fetus has a higher concentration due to different growth and metabolic rates. At the other end of the extreme, there is no placental transfer of plutonium or indium radionuclides.

Therefore, there seems to be an attempt by the mother to protect the fetus from some non-physiological elements and radionuclides.

Streffer: We need more data on this. We have identified some processes that eliminate radionuclides from the fetus. In the case of radiocaesium, for example, active transport is possible because the concentration in the fetus can be double that of the mother. For iodine, diffusion alone is involved when the thyroid is metabolically not active and the mother and fetus have roughly equal concentrations. However, as soon as the thyroid becomes active, the fetus takes up iodine rapidly. Therefore, these situations are complex, and they differ both between radionuclides and for the same radionuclide depending on its chemical form, as well as on the developmental stage.

Paretzke: You showed data for the number of cases as a function of dose. Some cases that were previously considered not exposed were reclassified into having been exposed to 1.5 Gy, which is a considerable exposure. What was the reason for this previous significant mis-classification?

Streffer: This difference can be explained on the two dosimetry systems TCD65 and DS86. The total number of cases was the same. The re-grouping from the TCD65 to the DS86 system causes a shift of some cases from the lower dose to the higher dose range.

Goldman: It is interesting that the DS86 dose model is probably bound to be changed once more because it now appears to be more like the older TCD65 model.

Streffer: I would like to mention a few aspects concerning this with respect to Down's syndrome. There were two cases of Down's syndrome in this time period (eight to 15 weeks postconception). If these are removed from the data set, which is justifiable because irradiation has not caused Down's syndrome in these cases (by irradiation eight to 15 weeks postconception no genetic effect was possible), a different dose–response curve is obtained. There is a threshold level of 0.40 Gy for all the cases, with a 95% confidence interval of 0.00–0.56 Gy. Therefore, a dose–response curve without a threshold is possible. However, if the Down's syndrome cases are removed, the threshold increases to 0.46 Gy and the 95% confidence interval is 0.23–0.61 Gy, so that a threshold is now possible. I would like to do a similar analysis of those people who were most contaminated after the Chernobyl accident to determine whether there is an analogous effect.

Goldman: But very few fetuses received a dose which was that large.

References

Cleaver JE 1968 Defective repair replication of DNA in xeroderma pigmentosum. Nature 218:652–656

Stewart A, Kneale GW 1970 Radiation dose effects in relation to obstetric X-rays and childhood cancer. Lancet 7658:1185–1188

UNSCEAR 1993 Sources and effects of ionizing radiation. United Nations Scientific Committee on the Effects of Atomic Radiation. United Nations, New York, p 139

Yoshimoto Y, Kato H, Schull WJ 1988 Risk of cancer among children exposed *in utero* to the bomb radiation. Lancet II:665–669

Late somatic health effects

Herwig G. Paretzke

GSF, Institut für Strahlenschutz, Ingolstädter Landstrasse 1, 85764 Neuherberg, Germany

Abstract. This chapter reviews the risks of radiation-induced cancer for the dose range likely to occur after releases of radionuclides into the environment. Epidemiological evidence from exposed workers and the atomic bomb survivors of Hiroshima and Nagasaki is surveyed. Influences on such risk functions of individual related quantities (e.g. age, sex, nationality, time since exposure and organs exposed) and of radiation modality-related quantities (e.g. dose, dose rate and radiation quality) are also briefly discussed.

1997 Health impacts of large releases of radionuclides. Wiley, Chichester (Ciba Foundation Symposium 203) p 167–177

Large releases of radionuclides into the environment can lead to populations being exposed to large collective doses of radiation. The maximum individual exposures are likely to decrease approximately linearly with the inverse distance from the source but the number of people exposed by a passing cloud increases approximately proportionally to the square of the distance. Therefore, most individual doses resulting from such a release will be small, i.e. of the order of magnitude of the annual natural and medical radiation exposure or small multiples thereof. These doses will mainly be delivered at small doses rates, i.e. over days, weeks or months.

Human experiences and experimental animal studies indicate that under these conditions the radiological consequences of exposures may be mainly late somatic health effects such as the induction of leukaemia and solid tumours. At these low doses and dose rates it is presently not possible to estimate human risks with reasonable accuracy directly from statistically significant data derived from the analysis of previous experience. This is because: (1) even in the absence of ionizing radiation the same health defects (cancers and leukaemias) are frequently the cause of death (ca. 15–25% of the total mortality is due to these causes); (2) these spontaneous probabilities show regional and temporal variations that are large compared to the assumed additional, radiation-related probabilities; and (3) it is currently not possible to identify the likely cause (e.g. smoking or previous irradiation with ionizing radiation) of a particular individual cancer or leukaemia.

The estimates used for the quantification of the corresponding health risks at low doses and dose rates must therefore be based on a series of extrapolating assumptions on, for example, shapes of specific dose–response curves and time-to-effect functions, distributions of sensitivities in the population, the transfer of risks derived from epidemiological studies in one particular region of the world to other populations, age and sex dependencies, and influences of radiation quality and dose rate.

This chapter will discuss: (1) the epidemiological evidence analysed for additional cases of cancer and leukaemias at low doses and dose rates in working environmental conditions; (2) the consequences of acute, higher dose irradiations due to the atomic bombings of Hiroshima and Nagasaki; and (3) the influences of individual- and radiation modality-related factors.

Epidemiological evidence for late effect risks of low dose and low dose rate exposures

In the context of large releases of radionuclides into the environment and of assessing their possible late somatic health effects it is reasonable to consider first epidemiological human studies investigating the mortality patterns of groups exposed to similar low levels of radiation at similar low dose rates. Such exposure conditions are found, for example, in the natural radiation environment, in areas of elevated fallout from previous atmospheric atomic bomb tests and in work places with levels of increased irradiation due to the presence of technical radiation sources (e.g. in nuclear facilities or in medicine) or to the technological enhancement of natural radiation exposures (e.g. in underground mines). Comprehensive overviews on the present knowledge in this field are given in UNSCEAR (1994) and Cox et al (1995).

Because of the reasons given above, however, such studies generally suffer from lack of statistical power and from the influence of confounding factors: in most studies hardly any excess cases are found at all. Therefore, at present, the quantitative low dose risk estimates for somatic late effects used in radiation protection are based on extrapolations of results from studies with higher statistical significance of persons exposed to high doses at high dose rates (see below). Nevertheless, it may be worthwhile to compare the regions of confidence of results from both types of studies using certain model assumptions (e.g. a linear no-threshold hypothesis of dose–response curves).

Regarding the possible effects of natural radiation exposures, in China the cancer rates found in populations living in two areas with different natural radiation backgrounds were compared by Wei et al (1990), particularly with respect to regional leukaemia rates. The results did not indicate significant differences between the rates in these two areas. Similar conclusions were drawn by Wang et al (1990a), who examined the prevalence of thyroid diseases and, in particular, of nodules (with may be linked to the later appearance of thyroid tumours) among women living in high background areas (about 140 mGy cumulative doses to the thyroid at age 50, about one-third of which were received during the sensitive period of childhood) compared to those living in areas with normal radiation levels (about 50 mGy dose to the thyroid).

However, in the high background areas there was significant evidence for higher levels of chromosome aberrations (without any obvious health consequences).

Cohen has published several papers on the geographical correlations between regional lung cancer rates in the USA and the average indoor radon concentrations (Cohen 1990, 1994, Cohen & Colditz 1994). He found no, or even a negative, correlation between these cancer rates and regional radon concentrations. However, Greenland & Robins (1994), Stidley & Samet (1994) and Piantadosi (1994) shed some general concern on the analytical usefulness of the statistical form of such a ecological study for radiation risk analysis, and they recommend other types of study designs (e.g. those based on individual exposure and effect data rather than average regional data). Therefore, no significant, quantitative conclusions can be drawn with respect to the health risks from radionuclides in the environment.

Several studies have investigated the possible health effects of irradiation, using geographical and temporal correlations and trend analyses, from global fallout radionuclides emitted into the environment by previous atmospheric tests of atomic weapons. In several of these studies, for example in the Nordic countries (Darby et al 1992) and in Utah, USA (Stevens et al 1990), a weak association between dose to the bone marrow and childhood leukaemia was found, which was consistent with the BEIR V (1990) leukaemia risk model.

Elevated levels of exposure to ionizing radiation have been found at particular work areas in the nuclear industry and in medicine, and in some countries (e.g. China, the USA and UK) studies have been performed with respect to the possible effects of these irradiations. In the medical area, radiologists and other medical X-ray workers have been exposed to high doses (often above 1 Gy), although their personal effective dose is difficult to determine retrospectively. Smith & Doll (1981), Matanoski et al 1984 and Wang et al (1990b) report increased risks among these medical groups in the UK, USA and China, respectively, for all types of cancer and for leukaemia. However, because of the uncertain dose estimations such data cannot be used for quantitative radiation risk assessment.

Gilbert et al (1993) studied the patterns of cancer and leukaemia rates in about 45 000 American nuclear workers at Oak Ridge, Rocky Flats and Hanford, but they found no significant effect of dose on these rates. Nevertheless, within large confidence limits, these data were found to be consistent with the present risk estimates for the Japanese atomic bomb survivors mentioned below. Some evidence of increased multiple myeloma risks with increasing dose was also observed.

Cancer mortality of about 95 000 British nuclear workers as a function of occupational dose has been analysed by Kendall et al (1992) in a study based on the UK National Registry for Radiation Workers, who received a mean lifetime dose at the work place of about 34 mSv (with about 8000 employees with occupational doses above 100 mSv); the total collective dose was 3198 Sv. The lifetime risk found for all malignant neoplasms, when a linear no-threshold and constant relative risk model was used for extrapolation, had a positive slope with dose (but not significantly) of $0.04 \, \text{Sv}^{-1}$ with 90% confidence interval limits of less than 0.0 and 0.6. For leukaemia, however, a statistically significant positive trend with dose was found ($P = 0.03$) and with a BEIR V type extrapolation model a central estimate risk for leukaemia induction of $0.0076\ \mathrm{Sv}^{-1}$ was derived. The 90% confidence limits here were both positive (0.0007 and 0.024). Also, these British data are consistent with the risk estimates based on the epidemiological conclusions for the acute irradiation of the survivors of Nagasaki and Hiroshima.

The International Agency for Research on Cancer published a multinational joint study on cancer risks among radiation workers in the USA, UK and Canada (IARC 1994). This study reported a significant increase of leukaemia risks with dose (excess relative risk of $2.2\ \mathrm{Sv}^{-1}$ with 90% confidence limits of 0.1 and 5.7); for all other cancers together the trend with dose was negative (but not statistically significantly), although the upper limit of the 90% confidence interval again was consistent with the Japanese data showing an excess relative risk of $0.39\ \mathrm{Sv}^{-1}$ (with 90% confidence limits of 0.32 and 0.46). This study will be continued and extended to several hundred thousand workers (Cardis et al 1992).

Because of the large areas of confidence of risk estimates based on the analysis of such data, they cannot be used alone for the assessment of health risks from ionizing radiation at low doses. This might change in the future if methods of molecular epidemiology are able to identify the possible causal origin of a given individual tumour.

Epidemiological evidence for late effect risks among the atomic bomb survivors

The epidemiological data of the survivors of the atomic bombings at Hiroshima and Nagasaki 50 years ago represent the most important source of information on the health risks of exposure to ionizing radiation (at high dose rate and of mainly low linear energy transfer). Ron et al (1994) and Thompson et al (1994) recently published updated data sets for the general cancer incidence and cancer mortality for the cohort of the life span study which includes about 93 000 survivors using the dosimetry system of 1986 and a constant neutron relative biological effectiveness of 10. Both sets clearly show an increased risk for all solid tumours as a group as well as for cancers of the bladder, breast, colon, liver, lung, ovary and stomach; the incidence data also show significant increases for some skin tumours and thyroid cancer. No significant excess risks were reported for either the cancer incidence or cancer mortality of the cervix, uterine corpus, gall bladder, kidney, larynx, pancreas, prostate and rectum. When summing up all risks for solid tumours occurring during the period 1950–1987 an excess relative risk for cancer mortality of $0.45\ \mathrm{Sv}^{-1}$ (with 90% confidencce limits of 0.3 and 0.6) and about a 50% higher value for the cancer incidence of $0.63\ \mathrm{Sv}^{-1}$ (with 90% confidence limits of 0.52 and 0.74) was derived. The respective values for the excess absolute risks are 11.1 ($10^4\ \mathrm{PYSv})^{-1}$ with 90% confidence limits of 8.4 and 14.0 for the cancer mortality and 29.7 ($10^4\ \mathrm{PYSv})^{-1}$ for the cancer incidence.

These data are based on a large population under observation (86 309) and on many cancer mortality cases (6887 observed, 6581 expected). However, when those $6887 - 6581 = 306$ excess cases are split up according to the rules of epidemiology and medicine into cohorts for the two cities, both sexes, age at exposure, time after exposure, dose group and cancer sites, it becomes evident that it is difficult (if not impossible), even with this extremely valuable data set, to estimate accurately the shape of organ-specific radiation risk functions at low doses without making many explicit or implicit assumptions. The situation is only somewhat better for the 75 excess leukaemia incidence cases, since the aspect of time extrapolation plays a minor role here and the smaller sub-classification dilutes these cases to a lesser extent.

Using a linear no-threshold theory and a reduction factor of two to account for the assumed lower effectiveness of small doses delivered at low dose rates, the ICRP (1990) has derived from the data of Shimizu et al (1990) for these atomic bomb survivors a lifetime cancer mortality risk of $0.04 \, \mathrm{Sv}^{-1}$ (90% confidence limits of 0.03 and 0.05) and a leukaemia risk of $0.004 \, \mathrm{Sv}^{-1}$ (90% confidence limits of 0.003 and 0.0055). These risk values for somatic late effects after irradiation with ionizing radiation are widely used.

Conclusion

Presently, there is no scientific expectation that from epidemiological data alone one will be able to assess late-effect radiation risks in the regime of normal radiation protection without many assumptions on the shape of the dose-effect curves, the effects of radiation quality, age at exposure, sex and time since exposure, for example. However, important co-ordinated scientific efforts are underway in applied radiation protection research (funded, for example, by the European Union) to describe quantitatively radiation carcinogenesis in a mechanistic, testable way so that in the future this shortcoming may be overcome. Because of the many contributing steps in the induction of neoplastic changes by radiation interaction with biological objects, the widely unknown processes during subsequent promotion and of the conversion into more malignant cells and final progression into a detectable tumour it is not likely that these scientific effort will soon lead to solid, quantitative estimations of late somatic risk functions at low doses. Until then, it will be advisable to use the risk estimates recommended by the United Nations Scientific Committee on the Effects of Atomic Radiation and the International Commission on Radiological Protection. However, it should be kept in mind that small doses of radiation alone apparently cannot produce large probabilities for adverse health effects. If this were so, these effects could be observed more clearly and subsequently analysed for a better risk quantification. On the other hand, the lack of statistical evidence of contributions of radiation to adverse health effects in epidemiological data should not be misinterpreted as evidence for the lack of such effects.

References

BEIR V 1990 NAS/NRC Committee on Biological Effects of Ionizing Radiation. V. Health effects of exposure to low levels of ionizing radiation. National Academy Press, Washington DC

Cardis E, Esteve J, Armstrong BK 1992 Meeting recommends international study of nuclear industry workers. Health Phys 63:405–406

Cohen BL 1990 A test of the linear no-threshold theory of radiation carcinogenesis. Environ Res 53:193–220

Cohen BL 1994 In defense of ecological studies for testing a linear no-threshold theory. Am J Epidemiol 139:765–768

Cohen BL, Colditz GA 1994 Tests of the linear no-threshold theory for lung cancer induced by exposure to radon. Environ Res 64:65–89

Cox R et al 1995 Risk of radiation-induced cancer at low doses and low dose rates for radiation protection purposes. Documents of the NRPB, Vol 6, No 1

Darby SC, Olsen JH, Doll R et al 1992 Trends in childhood leukemia in the Nordic countries in relation to fallout from atmospheric nuclear weapons testing. Br Med J 304:1005–1009

Gilbert ES, Cragle DL, Wiggs LD 1993 Updated analyses of combined mortality data for workers at the Hanford site, Oak Ridge National Laboratory, and Rocky Flats Weapons Plant. Radiat Res 136:408–421

Greenland S, Robins J 1994 Ecological studies: biases, misconceptions, and counterexamples. Am J Epidemiol 139:747–760

IARC 1994 Direct estimates of cancer mortality due to low doses of ionising radiation: an international study. International Agency for Research on Cancer study group on cancer risk among nuclear industry workers. Lancet 344:1039–1043

ICRP 1990 Recommendations of the International Commission on Radiological Protection. Publication 60. Pergamon, Oxford

Kendall GM, Muirhead CR, Macgibbon BH et al 1992 Mortality and occupational exposure to radiation. 1st analysis of the National Registry for Radiation Workers. Br Med J 304:220–225

Matanoski GM et al 1984 Cancer risks in radiologists and radiation workers. In: Boice JD, Fraumeni JF (eds) Radiation carcinogenesis — epidemiology and biological significance. Raven, New York, p 83–96

Piantadosi S 1994 Ecological biases. Am J Epidemiol 139:761–764

Ron E, Preston DL, Mabuchi K, Thompson DE, Soda M 1994 Cancer incidence in atomic bomb survivors. 4. Comparison of cancer incidence and mortality. Radiat Res 137:98S–112S

Shimizu Y, Kato H, Schull WS 1990 Studies of the mortality of A-bomb survivors. 9. Mortality, 1950–1985. 2. Cancer mortality based on the recently revised doses (DS86). Radiat Res 121:120–141

Smith PG, Doll R 1981 Mortality from cancer among British radiologists. Br J Radiol 54:187–194

Stevens W, Thomas DC, Lyon JL et al 1990 Leukemia in Utah and radioactive fallout from the Nevada test site: a case control study. J Am Med Assoc 264:585–591

Stidley CA, Samet JM 1994 Assessment of ecologic regression in the study of lung cancer and indoor radon. Am J Epidemiol 139:319–322

Thompson DE, Mabuchi K, Ron E et al 1994 Cancer incidence in atomic bomb survivors. 2. Solid tumours, 1958–1987. Radiat Res 137:17S–67S

UNSCEAR 1994 Sources and effects of ionizing radiation. Publication E.94.IX.11. United Nations Scientific Committee on the Effects of Atomic Radiation, United Nations, New York

Wang J-X, Inskip PD, Boice JD et al 1990 Cancer incidence among medical diagnostic X-ray workers in China, 1950 to 1985. Int J Cancer 45:889–895

Wang Z et al 1990 Thyroid nodularity and chromosome aberrations among women in areas of high background radiation in China. J Nat Cancer Inst 82:478–485
Wei LX, Zha YR, Tao ZF et al 1990 Epidemiologic investigation of radiological effects in high background radiation areas of Yangjiang, China. Radiat Res 31:119–136

DISCUSSION

Roed: Why are people with ankylosing spondylitis seldom used to study the risk of cancer?

Paretzke: One reason is that they are seriously ill people who may respond to irradiation in a different way to healthy people.

Goldman: Ankylosing spondylitis is a disease of the spinal column, and the bone marrow in the spinal column is also irradiated, so there's always a possibility that there may be an interaction between the medical condition and the risk.

Paretzke: Also, they receive drugs, which may have an effect either on their health status or on their risks.

Streffer: Nevertheless, the United Nations Scientific Committee on the Effects of Atomic Radiation (UNSCEAR) risk analysis, which is the basis of the risk analysis also currently used by the International Commission on Radiological Protection (ICRP), includes the data from ankylosing spondylitis. It is mostly based on the life span study from Japan, but it also includes two other studies with irradiated populations: one of ankylosing spondylitis and the other of cervix carcinomas.

Aarkrog: Do the data from Hiroshima and Nagasaki also have a bias similar to that of ankylosing spondylitis? There must have been a tremendous somatic stress on these people, which may have had a linear relationship to the dose they received.

Paretzke: That's a good question and I do not have a good answer. However, we are at least aware of this problem. There are, in principle, two possible opposing scenarios. The first scenarios is that of the 'survival of the fittest', i.e. those who survived these lethal explosions and the psychosomatic stress afterwards are much fitter than the average population. The risk factors derived from the later fate of these fit people may be too low for application to the average, less fit person. The second scenario is that the surviving exposed people might have been weakened by the traumas of the explosion, so that they became more sensitive to later health burdens. The risk factors derived from such a weakened population might be too low for application to normal, resistant people. The normal pattern of mortality in this population has been studied carefully. So far, nothing unusual about their life spans has been found. Therefore, I believe it is reasonable to treat them as average people and to use the radiation risk factors derived from their mortality statistics for other normal populations.

Roed: How does the low dose group compare to this group?

Paretzke: The individuals exposed to less than 50 mSv were about 2 km or more away from the 'ground zero' detonation point. Most of the houses within this distance were blown away and the whole city was largely destroyed within seconds.

Frissel: I would like to ask Herwig Paretzke if it is possible to use his model the other way round, i.e. to calculate how many million people are required in epidemiological studies before any conclusions can be drawn.

Paretzke: This could be done in principle but it's not particularly useful. This is because the larger the sample size in an epidemiological study the more heterogeneous the population and the larger the error bars of derived risks for individual sensitivities. This situation does not occur for laboratory mice, which are relatively homogeneous because of inbreeding. In this case it would be possible and meaningful to increase the sample size, but then one would have the problems of extrapolating the risks from mice to men.

Streffer: The population of West Germany is 60 million. The 95% confidence interval for accumulated cancer mortality during 75 years of life in Germany is higher than the irradiation risk of 100 mSv. In order to reach a radiation risk higher than this 95% confidence interval, a dose of 200 mSv is required, which shows the difficulty demonstrating such small radiation effects.

Herwig Paretzke showed some data on the incidence of leukaemia in exposed workers. The risk factors for leukaemia are about the same for the exposed workers and for those in Hiroshima and Nagasaki, but the situations are different, i.e. acute versus chronic exposure. In addition, different age groups were studied, i.e. adult workers and children.

Paretzke: If the numerical values for the late effect risk factors derived from the atomic bomb survivors and the nuclear workers in Great Britain are compared, it is merely accidental that they agree so well without the use of a dose rate reduction factor. However, I wouldn't draw the conclusion that this proves we should not use the dose rate reduction factor of 2.0 for low dose rates. The actual error margins in the case of the nuclear workers are much too large for this.

From the atomic bomb survivors we can derive a leukaemia risk factor of 0.4% per Sv, with 95% confidence limits of 0.30 and 0.55, if we use a dose rate reduction factor of 2.0. The radiation workers have a risk factor that is twice as large. However, their error margin is large, indicating that we should not focus on the factor itself but on its 95% confidence limits. Both confidence limits (of the nuclear workers and of the bomb survivors) overlap completely, which indicates consistency. The data on the American nuclear workers show that the collective dose of these 36 000 workers was only about one-tenth of the atomic bomb survivors and one-third of the British nuclear workers. The slopes of their dose–effect curves for leukaemias and solid tumours were negative and the upper 95% confidence intervals agree with the risk factors that the ICRP uses. This means that both data sets are consistent with the present risk estimates. I wouldn't draw any further conclusions from them.

Whicker: We often do hypothetical risk estimates for people exposed to hypothetical clean-up operations. We look at the entire sequence of transport through the food-chain, the dosimetry and the final risk estimates. In your opinion where does the greatest uncertainty lie?

Paretzke: With the risk estimates. This is because the estimated doses that you obtain are usually less than 10 mSv. Presently, we don't know whether such a dose causes cancer or not. This is often forgotten when such dose assessments are performed and used to calculate risks.

Whicker: It may be worthwhile to put our resources into those areas in which the greatest uncertainties lie. I have been more confident to date of the dose–risk uncertainties than of the transport uncertainties.

Paretzke: This is why a research project has been set up in the European Community to try to develop a quantitative model for low dose effects. In this project we would like to find out, for example, whether one single photon absorbed by a human body can cause cancer with a finite probability. This is an essential question because if such an interacting photon does not have a finite probability then our current 'linear, no-threshold' approach to somatic late effect risks might be seriously wrong.

Goldman: One of the problems with the low dose rate factor is that as this factor increases, so the correction factors for the confounding sociological, geological and genetic factors also increase. In an empirical, practical sense the Japanese data probably represent the limit of an epidemiological study. Another way to look at this is that several attempts have been made to compare the natural background radiations in different countries — such as France, China, Brazil and India — and there are no differences in the correlations between the incidences of cancer and the levels of background radiation. A few years ago in the USA the average background radiation for each state in the country was plotted against the total cancer mortality rate, and there was a negative correlation. This was explained by the observation that although the western, more mountainous regions had a higher background radiation, the populations in those areas had a large percentage of non-smoking Mormon people. Therefore, one must exercise caution when looking at simple correlations. The conventional wisdom is that perhaps 1% of cancer mortality is associated with natural background radiation, and until we obtain the mechanistic answer this is probably the best estimate that we'll have.

Paretzke: I would like to ask Christian Streffer a question about the linear dose–response curve for brain damage. Is it possible that low level radiation has an effect on the future intelligence of exposed fetuses and embryos?

Streffer: From a mechanistic point of view, it is unlikely. It is certainly a multicellular effect because many cells have to be damaged in order to result in mental retardation. It's not yet clear, at least from the epidemiological data, that such a threshold exists. Therefore, I would like to have more experimental data.

Goldman: If you do a brain scan you can observe that parts of the cerebrum are damaged in these high dosed, severely mentally retarded children.

Streffer: Three biological processes are affected by irradiation: cell proliferation, migration of the cells that form the cortex and natural cell death.

Roed: One could imagine that if many of the factors that increase susceptibility are present, then only a small input is sufficient to cause brain damage itself. This may result in a linear dose–response curve.

Streffer: A Gaussian distribution of intelligence has been discussed. One could imagine a shift in the dose–response to make it linear but at the moment, from a mechanistic point of view, a dose–response curve without a threshold is only possible if the brain damage is caused by a defect in only one cell, and this is apparently not the case. We don't yet have enough epidemiological data, and therefore all we can do is to extrapolate from animals to humans. However, it's difficult to extrapolate for intelligence, although we can do some extrapolations for brain capacity.

Renn: If one multiplies the risk potency factors for radon by the number of people exposed to different levels of radon and then adds this to the number of people who develop lung cancer from smoking, one obtains a number of expected lung cancer cases that is 30% over the number of actual lung cancer cases in the USA. Is this an indication that our models are too optimistic or that cigarette smoking is not as bad as we think? Alternatively, perhaps we should take the lower boundary of the confidence interval in order to explain this overshoot of the actual statistical data. Can anyone comment on this?

Paretzke: The cases who are smokers and develop lung cancer automatically include smokers who are exposed to radon.

Renn: But even if the interactive effects are removed, several sources claim that you still will end up with a value of more than 100%.

Paretzke: There are calculations that give this result but they are necessarily incorrect. In radiation protection we have to improve our respiratory tract model used in these calculations and dosimetric concepts. But this will take some time.

Goldman: It's also possible that the radon measurements are too high. Another relevant observation is that the lungs of smokers and non-smokers are not identical in terms of thickness of the mucosal wall, and this influences the range of α particles and the microdose distribution to critical cells.

Streffer: It has been shown in experimental systems, not on cancer induction but on cell damage, that interaction between two toxic agents is very much dependent on the dose.

Paretzke: Smoking can also produce a protective effect in the environment in that it produces aerosols that increase the deposition of radon daughter products attached to aerosols. Therefore, the inhalation of these daughter products is less likely. Secondly, α particles are somewhat shielded by the thicker mucosal layer of smokers and are therefore less likely to reach the basal cells and cause an initiating cancer effect. However, smoking can also have a synergistic effect with ionizing radiation. At present, we don't know whether we are dealing with additive effects, multiplicative effects or combinations thereof.

Goldman: There is another confusing aspect of extrapolating epidemiology. If one looks carefully at the Japanese atomic bomb survivor data, above an acute dose of 5 Gy most people were killed, whereas below 0.5 Gy there were few 'excess' cancer deaths (Shimizu et al 1987). Therefore, an extrapolation of these data to two to three orders of magnitude lower, which is the ball-park we are concerned with here, can produce large variations in the way the curve is drawn. In addition, the animal studies that have no uncertainty, at least about the dose, generate large uncertainties when they are extrapolated to humans (Thompson & Mahaffey 1986).

Paretzke: But this reduction of the effect with decreasing dose rates is not observed for low total doses. For example, in the mice data of Thompson & Mahaffey (1986), when the total dose was less than 0.2 Gy, the shortening of the mouse life span was found to be dependent only on the dose and not on the dose rate. We also have to be careful because in some experiments 100% of the animals finally develop a tumour. In this case, the only observable difference is a shift in the latency period, i.e. in the time when they develop a tumour. If one extrapolates the steepness of the dose–response curve, e.g. for osteosarcoma induction in beagles or rats, one may end up with something similar to an effective threshold. But this is mainly seen in experiments when the final tumour incidence is 100%. At lower doses the maximum incidence may only be 30%, for example, and in this case there is no clear evidence of a dose rate effect.

References

Shimizu Y, Kato H, Schull W, Preston D, Fujita S, Pierce D 1987 comparison of risk coefficients for site-specific cancer mortality based on the DS86 and T65DR shielded kerma and organ doses. Technical Report TR 12–87, Radiation Effects Research Foundation, Hiroshima, Japan

Thompson RC, Mahaffey JA 1986 Life-span radiation effects studies in animals: what can they tell us? United States Department of energy, CONF-830951 (DE87000490), National Technical Information Service, US Department of Commerce, Springfield, VA

Retrospective radiation dose assessment: an overview of physical and biological measures of dose

Marvin Goldman

Department of Radiological Sciences, University of California, 1122 Pine Lane, Davis, CA 95616–1729, USA

Abstract. Models to estimate population doses from environmental measurements, dietary radioactivity and lifestyle characteristics are useful for populations but difficult to apply accurately to an individual within the population. Individual biological and radiation dosimetry is limited to small numbers of persons and thus has limitations when considering larger groups or populations. Current direct biological indicators of dose are generally limited to doses above 0.1 Gy. New advances in improving the accuracy and sensitivity of these methods offer the promise of validating population estimates and specifying variance in individual doses. An integration of the two approaches will provide the support for more accurate radiation epidemiology and risk assessment.

1997 Health impacts of large releases of radionuclides. Wiley, Chichester (Ciba Foundation Symposium 203) p 178–187

Radiation dose reconstruction has become a significant environmental sciences speciality over the past decade. Models to integrate limited radiological measurements have been developed and are being validated and improved. For external exposures, our main tools are computer simulations of radiation output from a source term, be it the atomic bombs dropped on Japan or a hospital fluoroscope. Validation without actually duplicating the exposure conditions leaves a level of uncertainty that is difficult to reduce. The second major class of radiation dose reconstructions relates to those doses absorbed as a consequence of radionuclide intake. Here too, uncertainties exist as to the exact dosage quantity and quality, and pharmacokinetic behaviours in an individual or population are usually not available. I wish to restrict my remarks to this latter case, but I also realize that some of what I have to say may be germane to external exposure problems.

Simply stated, my thesis is that the reconstruction of doses from the outside inward can be assisted by personal biological radiation dosimetry from the inside out. I believe that the case can be made for the fact that deficiencies and limitations of environmental and biological dosimetry approaches are in different dimensions, and that the strengths of one can assist in reducing the weaknesses in the other. Ideally, an integration of biological and environmental dosimetry for the same case will be synergistic and the resultant collective uncertainty will be minimized. This is particularly true of low doses, where the sensitivity and detection limits of available techniques are stretched to their utmost. For radionuclide-related dose reconstruction, environmental measurements of concentrations and pathways are infrequently sufficient to determine accurately the quantity potentially taken in by an individual within a population. The sum of the appropriate biological, demographic and environmental factors generates the consequent dose estimate. In the best of all worlds, the findings might be confirmed by actually measuring excreta, body-burdens and/or biological indicators of radiation damage. We have rarely been able to realize this ideal because those exposed may have had doses that were below the sensitivity threshold for the available techniques.

I would like to review some of these techniques and present an argument for increased research and development of biological indicators that may provide more sensitive output. To keep this in perspective, I feel that there is an urgent need for improvement and advances in the environmental tools as well as for biological dosimeters. A host of sophisticated computer programs now provide a platform for rapid integration of data and integrated output of results. Atmospheric and environmental transport models have continued their evolution to powerful tools. Remote sensing of biological indicators, such as infra-red reflection and emission signatures of radiation-damaged plants, are now available. Aerial surveys, yielding planar spatial isoconcentration gradients of surface contamination, are being improved by integrating global-positioning systems with focal emission rate data. Faster processing and more sensitive, stable detectors are also providing improvements. On the ground, improved sampling techniques are providing concentration gradients and temporal and spatial profiles important for reconstructing prior situations. Thermoluminescent dosimetry of stable signals from radiation-exposed geological and biological samples add to our armament. All these techniques present opportunities for dynamic improvement. Added to these tools are the retrospective, historic description and documentation of events and measurements of past exposure-related information. At times, I am not too certain if there is adequate support and commitment for the development of further activities. I add my personal plea for a more integrated international programme to improve the sensitivity of techniques, to calibrate and certify the techniques, and to explore and develop new methods.

Biological dosimeters

The object of this overview is to indicate some important roles for biological indicators of radiation exposure in our overall planning for modern radiation retrospective dosimetry. These are either bioassays, i.e. direct physical measurements of radiation and radioactivity, or they are biological signals that are derived from living systems which record radiation effects.

Biological assays

Biological assays of radioactivity are simply collections of excreta from body burdens, the data from which, when inserted into pharmacokinetic models, provide an indirect estimate of the body burden and hence the associated radiation dose. This is particularly important for alpha-emitting radionuclides, whose emanations are too difficult or impossible to detect *in vivo*. Whole-body and partial-body counting techniques are especially sensitive for body burdens of gamma-emitting radionuclides. Energetic beta emitters can be assayed using bremsstrahlung counting and appropriate standards. Post-mortem tissue sampling, and in some cases tissue biopsy (e.g. tooth), can also provide direct input into body burden estimation.

Electron spin resonance

A renewed interest has developed for the use of electron spin resonance of biological crystals that have received radiation doses. Because of the long stability of the signal in exposed crystals, the technique has even been applied to dating of mastodon tusks, using the integrated natural background radiation signal over many thousands of years. More practically, it was used to measure the absorbed dose signal from the jaw of a survivor of the atomic bombing of Hiroshima 40 years ago. The crude device had poor sensitivity (i.e. 1 Gy) but it did demonstrate the feasibility of the method. For small chips of tooth enamel, a sensitivity of about 0.1 Gy is reported and a 10-fold improvement is quite possible.

I would like to make a plea here for a concentrated effort to exploit this technique to its limit, and to effectively engineer and develop both *in vivo* and *in vitro* methodologies that are internationally calibrated and accepted. My journeys through this technique over the past eight years have proven to me that many well-meaning scientists working competitively have not yet assembled the critical mass needed to achieve this goal in a reasonable time. For the dose reconstructions planned, as well as for accident management needs, there is no reason to continue in the present manner. In my view, this technique is as useful as the thermoluminescent dosimetry for personal and environmental dose documentation. This is one of my challenges to you.

Cellular markers

Cellular markers or indirect indicators of radiation dose are either cytological indicators or variations on measurement of somatic gene mutations. The advances in cell and molecular biology have not, in my opinion, been adequately carried over to the arena of biological dosimetry. Years ago we were promised an automated chromosome aberration-scoring device. We are still waiting for a dependable karyotype-scoring device. For the most part, the scoring of chromosomal aberrations is still done manually and tediously, as it was done some three decades ago. Where is the application of modern pattern recognition, so well developed for space applications but absent in microscopic assays? There have been a few heroic attempts to solve the problem, but it appears that there is no truly integrated heavy biological/engineering attack on the problem. The greatest interest for retrospective dosimetry is in stable chromosome translocation scoring, which is the least plentiful aberration. Therefore, it is all the more important to push this technology as far forward as is possible. In this case, sensitivity and accuracy are functions of the sheer number of cells that are scanned, and they are limited to the visual fatigue index of the scoring technician. This is another serious challenge for us to address.

The micronucleus test is useful, accurate and simple. It has a major drawback in that it does not distinguish between dividing and non-dividing cells, thus as an unstable aberration assay it is limited to short times after exposure and is not helpful in long-term retrospective dosimetry.

A newer cytogenetic tool to identify chromosomal translocations has now been developed. The use of fluorescence *in situ* hybridization (FISH) is now one of the more powerful techniques for identifying stable damage to chromosomes from radiation. The technique is complex and is at present limited to a few laboratories. It is costly and it remains to be seen if some automated modification will become available that can increase its applicability, efficiency and sensitivity to detect small radiation doses. It has sufficient promise though, such that I would encourage a quantum increase of multi-disciplinary expertise focused on this assay, especially in determining its ultimate sensitivity. This is my third challenge.

For several years, we have been presented with an array of somatic gene mutation techniques. One that has received much attention recently is the glycophorin-A assay, which uses a fluorescently labelled monoclonal antibody to measure the loss of an erythrocyte allele in irradiated people. It is purported to be a stable indicator, with lifelong persistence. I am not enough of a biochemist to go into great detail, but I am concerned that the technique has severe limitations as a reliable radiation biodosimeter. It does not appear to be reproducible within the same individual, even though millions of erythrocytes are measured in the assay. There seems to be a great variability among individuals exposed to the same dose, and there has not yet been a careful calibration using persons with known exposures. It is simple, relatively cheap and potentially useful, but only if it can be calibrated and validated.

As with the micronucleus test mentioned above, the HPRT mutation assay (hypoxanthine phosphoribosyltransferase mutations in T lymphocytes) is limited to short times after exposure. In addition, its signal fades rapidly. Another assay, the HLA-A (human leukocyte antigen A) assay is tedious, insensitive and not promising at the moment. The beta globulin test likewise offers some promise, but it is too early to state if this fluorescent antibody indicator of a single base change in haemoglobin can provide a practical tool. There may be other useful biodosimeter techniques in various stages of development.

Individual biological dosimetry: an integral part of radiation dose reconstruction

What is advocated here is the full utilization of these biomarkers as integral elements in future radiation dose reconstructions. What I have seen thus far is the occasional use of one or more assays, more as an afterthought than an integral part of the protocol. The reason that is usually put forth is that the techniques are too expensive and technology intensive, and they have insufficient radiation reliability and/or sensitivity. However, the limitations of environmental radiation dose reconstruction also entail significant uncertainties about the variables used in modelling, no matter how sophisticated the tool.

While we are improving the validation and calibration of these models, why not also put in the effort to render the biological tools more sensitive and reproducible? Incorporating statistically appropriate individual measurements in the reconstruction matrix can add a powerful dimension to our efforts at dose reconstruction. I envisage a time in the near future when there will be a convergence of these two approaches, with a resultant synergy of action that produces dose reconstructions with minimal uncertainty and maximal credibility. I can see where the strengths of each technology can assist in reducing the weaknesses of the other, which will help us to answer important questions about prior radiation exposures. Major resources are expended on epidemiology studies, with great emphasis on confounding factors — for example, on subtracting natural disease rates from the subject population. However, this emphasis on reducing uncertainties on the ordinate of the dose–effect relationship must be accompanied by an equal dedication to minimizing uncertainties about dose. Population estimates based solely on broad environmental models, although sensitive, can only be verified by the use of individual measurements. Despite almost a half century of work, estimates of individual doses in survivors of the atomic bombing of Japan are still uncertain. New biological dosimetry can, and is, helping us to reduce this uncertainty; and so it should be applied to the other populations that have been exposed to radiation. That is my final challenge to you.

Further reading

Akiyama M, Kyoizumi S, Hirai Y, Hakoda M, Nakamura N, Awa AA 1990 Studies on chromosome aberrations and HPRT mutations in lymphocytes and GPA mutation in erythrocytes of atomic bomb survivors. Prog Clin Biol Res 340:69C–80C

Albertini R, Castle KL, Borcherding WR 1982 T-cell cloning to detect the mutant 6-thioguanine-resistant lymphocytes present in human peripheral blood. Proc Natl Acad Sci USA 79:6617–6621

Anspaugh LR, Catlin RJ, Goldman M 1988 The global impact of the Chernobyl reactor accident. Science 242:1513–1519

Bender MA, Awa AA, Brooks AL et al 1988 Current status of cytogenetic procedures to detect and quantify previous exposures to radiation. Mutat Res 196:103–159

Boecker B, Hall R, Inn K 1991 Current status of bioassay procedures to detect and quantify previous exposures to radioactive materials. Health Phys (Suppl 1) 60:45–102

Chong TS, Hirouki D, Yoshiyuki N, Takao I, Kenga I, Hideo S 1989 ESR dating of elephant teeth and radiation dose rate estimation in soil. Int J Rad Appl Instrum A 40:1199–1202

Cremer T, Popp S, Emmerich P, Lichter P, Cremer C 1990 Rapid metaphase and interphase detection of radiation-induced chromosome aberrations in human lymphocytes by chromosomal suppression *in situ* hybridization. Cytometry 11:110–118

Eisert WG, Mendelsohn ML (eds) 1984 Biological dosimetry. Springer-Verlag, Berlin

Evans HJ 1988 Mutation cytogenetics: past, present and future. Mutat Res 204:355–363

Evans HJ, Lloyd DC (eds) 1978 Mutagen-induced chromosome damage in man. Edinburgh University Press, Edinburgh

Fenech M, Morley AA 1985 Measurement of micronuclei in lymphocytes. Mutat Res 147:29–36

Gesell TF, Voilleque PG (eds) 1990 Evaluation of environmental radiation exposures from nuclear testing in Nevada. Health Phys 59:501–762

Goldman M, Catlin R, Anspaugh LR 1987 Health and environmental consequences of the Chernobyl nuclear power plant accident. US Department of Energy Report DOE/ER-0332. Washington, DC

Hennequin C, Cosset JM, Cailleux PE et al 1989 Amylasemia: a biological marker for irradiation accidents?: preliminary results obtained at the Institut Gustave-Roussy and a review of the literature. Bull Cancer (Paris) 76:617–624

Ikeya M, Ishii H 1989 Atomic bomb and accident dosimetry with ESR: natural rocks and human tooth *in vivo* spectrometer. Int J Rad Appl Instrum A 40:1021–1027

Janatipour M, Trainer KJ, Kutlaca R et al 1988 Mutations in human lymphocytes studied by an HLA selection system. Mutat Res 198:221–226

Langlois RG, Bigbee WL, Jensen RH 1986 Measurements of the frequency of human erythrocytes with gene expression loss phenotypes at the glycophorin A locus. Hum Genet 74:353–362

Lushbaugh C, Eisele G, Burr W, Hubner K, Wacholz B 1991 Current status of biological indicators to detect and quantify previous exposures to radiation. Health Phys (suppl 1) 60:103–109

Mendelsohn ML 1990 New approaches for biological monitoring of radiation workers. Health Phys 59:23–28

Mettler FA, Kelsey CA, Ricks RC 1990 Medical management of radiation accidents. CRC Press, Boca Raton, FL

Müller W-U, Streffer C 1991 Biological indicators for radiation damage. Int J Radiat Biol & Relat Stud Phys Chem & Med 94:863–873

Nakajima T 1989 Possibility of retrospective dosimetry for persons accidently exposed to ionizing radiation using electron spin resonance of sugar and mother-of-pearl. Br J Radiol 62:148–153

Pasquier C, Masse R 1991 Biological dosimetry. Radioprotection (suppl) 26:155–297

Prosser JS, Moquet JE, Lloyd DC, Edwards AA 1988 Radiation induction of micronuclei in human lymphocytes. Mutat Res 199:37–45

Regulla DP, Deffner U 1989 Dose estimation by ESR spectroscopy at a fatal radiation accident. Int J Rad Appl Instrum Part A 40:1039–10433

Scheid W, Weber J, Traut H 1988 Chromosome aberrations induced in human lymphocytes by an X-radiation accident: results of a 4-year postirradiation analysis. Int J Radiat Biol & Relat Stud Phys Chem & Med 54:395–402

Seifert AM, Bradley WEC, Messing K 1987 Exposure of nuclear medicine patients to ionizing radiation is associated with rises in HPRT-mutant frequency in peripheral T lymphocytes. Mutat Res 191:57–63

Sposto R, Stram DO, Awa AA 1990 An investigation of random errors in the DS86 dosimetry using data on chromosome aberrations and severe epilation. TR 7-90. Radiation Effects Research Foundation, Hiroshima

Stram DO, Mizuno S 1989 Analysis of the DS86 atomic bomb radiation dosimetry methods using data on severe epilation. Radiat Res 117:93–113

Tates AD, Bernini LF, Natarajan AT et al 1989 Detection of somatic mutants in man: HPRT mutations in lymphocytes and hemoglobin mutations in erythrocytes. Mutat Res 213:73–82

Toohey R, Palmer E, Anderson L et al 1991 Current status of whole body counting as a means to detect and quantify previous exposures to radioactive materials. Health Phys (suppl 1) 60:7–42

Trask B, Vandenengh G, Pinkel D et al 1988 Fluorescence *in situ* hybridization to interphase cell nuclei in suspension allows flow cytometric analysis of chromosome content and microscopic analysis of nuclear organization. Hum Genet 78:251–259

Zoetelief J, Broerse JJ 1990 Dosimetry for radiation accidents: present status and prospects for biological dosimeters. Int J Radiat Biol & Relat Stud Phys Chem & Med 57:737–750

DISCUSSION

Lake: The electron spin resonance (ESR) technique has many advantages but wouldn't it be much more expensive to use *in vivo* than any of the other methods?

Goldman: Not necessarily. The machine is similar to a portable X-ray machine, so although it would cost several hundred thousand dollars to develop, once it was developed it could be reproduced for a few thousand dollars. The only technical points that are going to take some time and effort are getting the magnet and the resonance correct. It's one of my challenges to get the engineering and biological communities together to solve this.

Paretzke: Your sensitivity numbers are somewhat optimistic. We are working on this method but until now we haven't dared to state an *in vitro* estimate for doses less than 0.3 Gy with less than 100% error. Therefore, I'm doubtful as to whether one can make such low dose estimates *in vivo*. This is a dose regime where normal cytogenetic dosimetry isn't that inaccurate. There are well-established, cheaper methods that are already available today, although they may be somewhat slower.

Goldman: But technical improvements are possible. For example, most of the work on tooth enamel is done by grinding up a chip. However, if it is not ground up, but orientated in a certain way there is about a fivefold improvement in the signal-to-noise ratio (M. Derossier, personal communication 1990). I'm asking whether we can push this further. I'm not suggesting that we're necessarily at the limit.

Streffer: How much material would you need for ESR analysis?

Goldman: Not more than a milligram.

Balonov: You made many suggestions for biological dosimetry techniques. In your opinion, which of these is the most promising?

Goldman: The fluorescence *in situ* hybridization technique has the greatest potential because to date it has not been as fully automated as is conceivable. It's still a largely manual effort, and for many of these techniques, sensitivity is a function of how many things one can measure — for example, how many cells can be scored. Also, if it's an optical technique, fatigue may be a problem, so that a worker can only score perhaps 100–200 cells at a time. An automated technique would be able to score 10 000 cells reproducibly, which would be a vast improvement.

Bauchinger: Concerning the ESR dosimetry, is it possible to discriminate between high and low linear energy transfer effects, for example between alpha irradiation and gamma irradiation?

Goldman: I don't know the answer to this. The path length of alpha particles going into mineral would be very short, so there would be surface activation. One has to consider the ESR of the crystals within a layer of hydroxyapatite, so the alpha particle is not going to penetrate deeply and only the surface crystals will be exposed to them. Therefore, there will be the problem of a surface-to-volume correction.

Paretzke: Another problem will arise from potential internal contamination by strontium. In this case there will be radicals produced by the tooth internal dose as well as those produced by external irradiation. Trying to separate these measurements will be difficult.

Goldman: There may be an interesting biological solution in that tooth dentine will have a ^{90}Sr deposition pattern because it turns over.

Paretzke: But the resulting uncertainties in both contributions will be large.

Streffer: If alpha particles such as radon give a signal in the teeth then the method would be worthless because the doses on teeth from natural sources would be so high that they would cover up everything else.

Goldman: I'm not hopeful that the ESR technique could be used for radon.

Streffer: Can it give any indication about the dose rate?

Goldman: The technique is not dose rate sensitive. It gives information about the integral dose and not about the dose rate.

Bauchinger: Would a metal inlay in a tooth be a confounding factor of the dose estimation?

Goldman: Not necessarily. As long as the metal was half a millimetre away or so it probably wouldn't be a problem.

Paretzke: I would like to discuss this from a more philosophical point of view. If there is a large variability in the response of a biological indicator to a physical dose, this may be telling us that there is a biological variation in the response. Therefore, an objective physical quantity such as absorbed dose might be a less relevant quantity for subsequent risk assessment than a subjective, individual biological response.

Goldman: I understand the philosophical aspect, but in my opinion the ESR test is not useful for this particular set of questions; it is a physical not a biological indicator test. Some of the other tests have a greater capability of reducing the uncertainty about what the physical dose actually was. Once we determine this, we can then concentrate more on the variations in biological response, which is an area that is still embryonic.

Paretzke: Let us assume that a particular type of cancer has a strong causal relationship with a certain type of chromosome aberration. If the induction of this chromosome aberration at the same physical dose shows different yields in different persons due to intraspecies variation, then a measurement of the yield of chromosome aberrations most likely would be a more reasonable indicator of the subsequent individual risks of this type of tumour than the physical dose.

Goldman: I look upon these biological indicators as a measure of the initiating event. The data show that the progression to cancer involves an initiating event followed by a series of promoting steps, which incorporate such aspects as variability. For example, the ability to repair DNA is not identical in different individuals. The sum of each of the minor efficiency variations in exonucleases, endonucleases and other repair enzymes constitute our biological variability. Therefore, I would like to see a minimum variation in terms of the initiating events. As we learn more about the molecular biology of these sequential events, we are beginning to see that exposure does not equal risk. It's our best practical way of handling risk, but it does not represent risk. We need to know more about the rest of the biology that follows the initial physical event.

Bauchinger: You suggested that the glycophorin-A assay cannot be used as a lifetime dosimeter, but only for a maximum of two or three years. Can you tell us a little more about the glycophorin-A assay? Because some groups are trying to introduce this assay in Germany, even though they have no particular expertise in using it.

Goldman: I stumbled upon this evaluation whilst reading Langlois et al (1987). They looked at individual glycophorin-A measurements in the Japanese atomic bomb survivors and related them to their assigned radiation exposures. It was fortuitous that the pattern looked like a shotgun pattern. I haven't seen any more assessments of this assay, but I know that it has been done for other radiation patients.

Bauchinger: So you wouldn't recommend using this test?

Goldman: I wouldn't incorporate this as my standard technique until I tested it further. There are many people with known exposures, whom one could test. Also, half of the population only has one of these alleles, and the test is only good for those who have both.

Lake: These data are nine years old. There must surely be something more solid than this?

Bauchinger: The data are from a highly respected group. There are also some other data from the Lawrence Livermore Laboratory on Chernobyl clean-up workers, showing that variant cell frequencies have been stably expressed for seven years post-exposure. This indicates that the glycophorin-A assay may provide a means for a cumulative dose measurement (Jensen et al 1995).

Goldman: These data are not much better. They suffer from the same problem. It would be interesting to analyse the same 40 people from this test with the fluorescence *in situ* hybridization and ESR techniques because they represent independent checks. Furthermore, repeated analysis on the same individual doesn't give the same reading, so this is another problem. I don't want you all to feel that this is the final word. I am only asking you to be cautious when using these techniques.

References

Jensen H J, Langlois RG, Bigbee WL et al 1995 Elevated frequency of glycophorin-A mutations in erythrocytes from Chernobyl accident victims. Radiat Res 141:129–135

Langlois RG, Akiyama M, Kusunoki Y et al 1993 Analysis of somatic cell mutations at the glycophorin-A locus in atomic bomb survivors: a comparative study of assay methods. Radiat Res 136:111–117

Cytogenetic effects as quantitative indicators of radiation exposure

Manfred Bauchinger

Institut für Strahlenbiologie, GSF-Forschungszentrum für Umwelt und Gesundheit, Postfach 1129, D-85758, Oberschleissheim, Germany

Abstract. Scoring of dicentrics in metaphase preparations of human T lymphocytes is the method of choice for estimating individual whole-body doses of radiation exposure. A quantification of partial-body exposures or non-uniform distribution of the dose is more complicated but it can be achieved by using specific mathematical approaches. For retrospective biodosimetry, conventional scoring of dicentrics is less precise because these unstable aberrations are eliminated with time post-exposure. Symmetrical translocations are not selected against during mitotic division in the haematopoietic cell reproductive centres, so the frequencies of these stable aberrations are generally assumed to remain constant even for decades. They can now be analysed precisely by fluorescence *in situ* hybridization using whole chromosome-specific DNA probes (chromosome painting) with an α-satellite DNA probe for centromere detection. Based on *in vitro* calibration curves established with single or multicolour paints covering 4–22% of the total human genomic DNA content, scoring of translocations has been applied for dose reconstruction in smaller groups of atomic bomb survivors and victims of the Chernobyl and Goiania radiation accidents. However, prior to routine use, the method requires further validation. Such work includes the precise evaluation of the unexpectedly high frequency of complex exchanges ($\geqslant 3$ breaks in $\geqslant 2$ chromosomes) found both at $> 2\,\mathrm{Gy}$ doses of low linear energy transfer (LET) radiation and generally for high LET α-particles. Data on the long-term stability of translocations and the appearance of clonal aberrations, as well as improved measurements of the linear coefficient of standard calibration curves, are also required.

1997 Health impacts of large releases of radionuclides. Wiley, Chichester (Ciba Foundation Symposium 203) p 188–204

Accidental over-exposure to ionizing radiation requires a rapid and precise reconstruction of the absorbed dose and its distribution in the body in order to provide an early evaluation of radiological consequences, decisions for immediate medical treatment and data for risk analysis. Among various attempts of quantifying human radiation exposure, cytogenetic or biological dosimetry has proven reliable for estimating the dose to individuals and to population groups (for review see Bauchinger 1995a). In the initial phase of the major radiation accidents of Chernobyl, Ukraine (IAEA 1986a) and Goiania, Brazil (IAEA 1988), scoring of dicentrics and ring

188

chromosomes in peripheral blood lymphocytes was important for the selection of victims requiring either bone marrow transplantation (Chadwick & Gerber 1991) or specific individual care (Ramalho et al 1988). For retrospective dosimetry, chromosome analysis in its conventional form is less precise because unstable aberrations, such as dicentrics, are eliminated from the peripheral blood with time post-exposure (Buckton et al 1978). Fluorescence *in situ* hybridization (FISH) with whole chromosome-specific DNA probes (chromosome painting) can now be used as an alternative method for a rapid and precise scoring of symmetrical translocations and insertions (Pinkel et al 1986). These aberrations are commonly classified as stable because their frequencies do not appear to change with time. The technique is not yet fully standardized or validated, but it has the potential to be used even decades after the exposures. The main principles of both techniques will be demonstrated, and their reliability and limitations will be discussed.

Lymphocyte culture

Chromosome analyses are performed in T lymphocytes two days after the cell cultures have been stimulated to proliferate. Dicentrics alone are generally scored in conventional analyses. Sometimes ring chromosomes are also included, but their frequency is only about 5–10% of the numbers of dicentrics. In proliferating cells 50% of the dicentrics are lost during the first division post-irradiation; therefore, their frequency is underestimated in any quantitative analysis that does not use exclusively first cycle metaphases. This source of error can, however, be eliminated by the use of fluorescence plus Giemsa (FPG) harlequin staining after treating T lymphocyte cultures with 5-bromodeoxyuridine (BrdU), since a perfect discrimination between the first and later cell cycle metaphases is achieved.

Conventional chromosome analysis

The background frequency of dicentrics is low: it ranges between zero and 2.35×10^{-3} per cell (Bender et al 1988). In a control group of 79 individuals, 17 dicentrics (and five ring chromosomes) were found in 43 000 cells. This corresponds to a mean value of $0.40 \ (\pm 0.10) \times 10^{-3}$ dicentrics, with 95% confidence limits of 0.22 and 0.61 (Bauchinger 1995b).

   In vitro dicentric dose–response curves for relevant radiation qualities must be obtained for calibration purposes. Linear–quadratic ($Y = c + \alpha D + \beta D^2$, with c = control frequency) and linear ($Y = c + \alpha D$) dose–response relationships are generally obtained for low and high linear energy transfer (LET) radiations, respectively. Fitted coefficients of typical calibration curves are shown in Table 1. The differential biological effectiveness of the various radiation qualities is apparent in Fig. 1, which shows that high LET radiation is more efficient at producing dicentrics than low LET radiation.

TABLE 1   Fitted coefficients α and $\beta \pm$ S.E. of the dose–response curves $Y = \alpha D + \beta D^2$ for dicentrics (lines 1–5, conventional analysis, see Fig. 1) and translocations (lines 6 and 7, fluorescence *in situ* hybridization measurements, see Fig. 3) after *in vitro* exposure of human T lymphocytes to various radiation qualities

Radiation quality	$\alpha \pm S.E.\ (10^{-1}Gy^{-1})$	$\beta \pm S.E.\ (10^{-2}Gy^{-2})$
^{60}Co γ-rays, (0.017 Gy/min)	0.090 ± 0.400	4.17 ± 0.28
^{60}Co γ-rays, (0.5 Gy/min)	0.107 ± 0.041	5.55 ± 0.28
220 kV X-rays (0.5 Gy/min)	0.404 ± 0.030	5.98 ± 0.17
14.5 MeV (d+T) neutrons	1.790 ± 0.150	7.40 ± 1.39
Fission neutrons, $\bar{E}$ 1.6 MeV	3.690 ± 0.210	13.34 ± 1.73
^{137}Cs γ-rays	0.059 ± 0.043	1.67 ± 0.13
220 kV X-rays	0.094 ± 0.047	2.86 ± 0.30

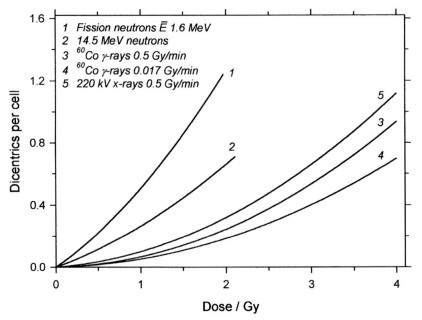

FIG. 1.   Linear, quadratic dose–response curves for dicentrics (conventional analysis) for the various radiation qualities indicated.

The induction of comparable yields of dicentrics in T lymphocytes irrespective of exposure *in vivo* or *in vitro* is a main prerequisite for using these calibration curves to estimate an individual's exposure. This has been proven for whole-body irradiation in animal experiments, and it could be confirmed for the therapeutic whole-body exposure of cancer patients to low LET radiation.

Biological dose estimates with uncertainties expressed as 95% confidence intervals can be obtained from the calibration curves, and they represent equivalent, uniform whole-body doses. The most reliable dose estimates can be obtained from recent, largely uniform, acute whole-body exposures. Individual external doses of low LET radiation in the region of 100 mGy can be reliably measured. The detection of lower acute doses or of accumulated doses from long-term exposures to low LET radiation, e.g. of the order of maximum permissible occupational limits (50 mGy), is less certain because the degree of induced aberration yields is small compared to the background frequency (for review see Bauchinger 1995b). Provided that a sufficiently large number of cells (depending on the background value of dicentrics, this is at least 20 000–30 000) is scored, exposures down to about 50 mGy may be detectable. However, this applies only for population groups.

Quantification of partial-body or non-uniform exposures is also difficult. Non-homogeneous exposure may result from a differential absorption of radiation in soft tissues and bones. As a consequence, fluctuations in local doses occur, leading to the differential exposure of T lymphocytes in variable volumes of the irradiated region of the body. This situation is complicated by the observation that, at any particular time, only 3–5% of the total T lymphocytes of a healthy young adult reside in the peripheral blood, with a mean residence time of about 20–30 min (Trepel 1975, 1976). In addition most of the T lymphocytes are stored in lymphatic tissues or other organs and may recirculate into the peripheral blood. Therefore, for a partial-body exposure, one is always dealing with irradiated and unirradiated populations of T lymphocytes. Particularly at high doses, various cellular reactions — such as reduced blast transformation, mitotic delay and interphase death — may lead to a preferential selection of heavily damaged cells. This explains why, despite extremely large doses, meaningful biological dose estimates sometimes cannot be obtained for accidental exposures involving small volumes, such as hands or fingers. In such cases, there are insignificant frequencies of chromosomal aberrations.

For larger partial-body exposures, mathematical–statistical analyses of chromosome aberration data can be performed to derive a dose estimate for the irradiated fraction of the body. This is more realistic than quoting a mean equivalent, uniform whole-body dose. It can be achieved by the 'contaminated Poisson' method of Dolphin (1969) or by the Q_{dr} method of Sasaki (1983), which are based on similar principles. For a detailed description of the mathematical procedures see (IAEA 1986b).

The first approach uses information on the intercellular distribution of dicentrics in the total number of scored cells. Following a uniform exposure of T lymphocytes to low LET radiation, dicentrics should be randomly distributed and follow a Poisson distribution, which is characterized by a variance equal to the mean. So-called over-dispersion, i.e. a variance greater than the mean, can be taken as an indication of non-uniform exposure. The fraction of irradiated T lymphocytes in the body and the mean dose can be obtained from the degree of the deviation from the Poisson distribution. Over-dispersion is generally observed for high LET radiation; therefore, this method is restricted to low LET radiation. A further limitation is that for local doses, which are too low to produce a sufficient number of cells containing several dicentrics, the frequency of irradiated cells exhibiting no aberrations (zero class of the Poisson distribution) cannot be estimated precisely. For statistical reasons, sufficiently high cell numbers are also required.

The alternative Q_{dr} method considers the frequency of dicentrics and rings only in cells containing dicentrics, ring chromosomes and acentric fragments. These cells have a selective disadvantage during cell proliferation and they are therefore termed unstable (C_u-cells). They belong to the irradiated fraction of T lymphocytes and, provided that they are analysed exclusively in their first division post-irradiation, they must have retained their initial chromosomal damage. The Q_{dr} value represents the expected frequency of dicentrics and ring chromosomes among the first division C_u-cells. It is dose dependent, but independent of dose homogeneity and of the dilution of damaged cells by undamaged cells originating either from unexposed parts of the

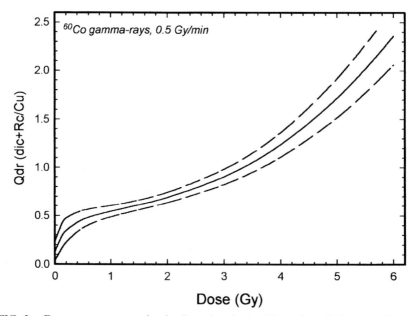

FIG. 2. Dose–response curve for the Q_{dr} value obtained from the radiation experiment 3 in Fig. 1 (^{60}Co γ-rays at 0.5 Gy/min). Dashed lines represent the limits of a 95% confidence interval. $Q_{dr} = Y_{dr}/(1-\exp(-Y_{dr}-Y_{ace}))$, where Y_{dr} and Y_{ace} represent the dose–response relationships for dicentrics (dic) plus ring chromosomes (Rc) and acentrics, respectively (conventional analysis). Cu, unstable cells.

body or from the cell reproductive centres. From a dose–response curve for Q_{dr} values (Fig. 2), generated from an *in vitro* experiment with ^{60}Co γ-rays (Bauchinger et al 1983), dose estimates can be derived for the irradiated part of the body. A reliable application of the Q_{dr} method requires, however, an observation of at least 20 C_u-cells. For a total of 1000 analysed cells, this corresponds to a dose of about 250 mGy.

Conventional scoring of dicentrics is also limited for assessing radiation doses of past exposures due to the temporal decline of cells containing unstable dicentrics. This limitation is relevant in the dose reconstruction of critical populations exposed to radioactive fallout depositions from the Chernobyl reactor accident in April 1986 and from the accident at the Mayak's separation plant near the village Kyshtym (Southern Ural) in September 1957. Various mathematical models describing the rate of this decline are available (Buckton 1983, Léonard et al 1988, Bauchinger et al 1989, Bogen 1993), and they can be used to correct for the post-exposure time-lapse when a dose reconstruction has to be performed from unstable aberration frequencies. However, the repopulation kinetics of the affected haematopoietic stem cell compartments is complex and reveals a considerable fluctuation. Thus, particularly for severe over-exposures, reasonable individual dose estimates sometimes cannot be obtained, or at least they may contain large uncertainties (Littlefield et al 1991). Provided that a sufficient number of C_u-cells can be found, the Q_{dr} method may also be used for dose reconstruction because the Q_{dr} value is independent on the time post-exposure. It would thus appear that the most reliable retrospective biological dosimetry can be expected from measuring yields of stable chromosome aberrations, such as symmetrical translocations and insertions, which are not eliminated with time post-irradiation. To date, these rearrangements have been analysed by chromosome banding, which is too laborious for routine use. However, they can now also be scored precisely by chromosome painting.

Chromosome painting

The FISH technique with composite whole chromosome-specific DNA probes provides uniform labelling of the homologues of a particular target chromosome along their entire length (chromosome painting). Probes labelled with various reporter molecules or directly fluorescently labelled probes can be used to paint single homologues or cocktails mostly consisting of two or three chromosomes in a single- or multi-colour fluorescence assay. Using a suitable counterstain for non-hybridized chromosome regions, structural rearrangements involving target chromosomes can be easily detected by their bi- or multi-colour fluorescence pattern. The simultaneous use of a degenerate α-satellite DNA probe facilitates a precise discrimination between translocations and dicentrics (Weier et al 1991, Bauchinger et al 1993). Protocols providing a cell cycle-controlled analysis by combing BrdU/FPG harlequin staining/FISH technologies are also available (Kulka et al 1995).

Several data on radiation-induced chromosome aberrations showed that FISH painting also revealed complex exchanges ($\geqslant 3$ breaks in $\geqslant 2$ chromosomes). Their frequency was unexpectedly high both at > 2 Gy doses of low LET radiation (Simpson & Savage 1994, 1995) and generally for high LET α-particles (Griffin et al 1995). Beyond this a substantial proportion of apparently simple exchanges were complex derived. These findings complicate an appropriate conversion of complex exchange patterns into translocation yields, which is required for the quantification of the total actual damage. Two recently developed nomenclature systems — complex exchange/ break number analysis (Savage & Simpson 1994); and PAINT (Tucker et al 1995a), which analyses any aberrant chromosome configuration — may be used to overcome these problems. However, both of these require validation for routine use.

Like conventional biodosimetry, standard translocation calibration curves must be generated (Fig. 3 and Table 1). Linear–quadratic curves, particularly those including low doses (about 100 mGy), are scarce. In addition, existing low LET radiation data do not provide a certain value for the α coefficient. Compared to conventional dicentric background data, far higher translocation frequencies (up to 10-fold) and a higher interindividual variability (0–4 translocations versus 0–1 dicentrics/1000 cells per case) have been observed with FISH. As a consequence, more cells must be scored to reduce the α coefficient uncertainties, and larger control groups must be examined to obtain more information on the potential influence of population variables — such as age, smoking, clastogenic environmental chemicals and medical drugs — on the

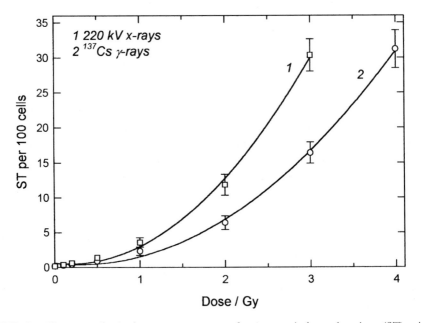

FIG. 3.   Linear, quadratic dose–response curves for symmetrical translocations (ST) using fluorescence *in situ* hybridization (painting of chromosomes 1, 4 and 12) for ^{37}Cs γ-rays and 220 kV X-rays. Error bars show S.E.M.

background level of stable translocations. This information is essential for a reliable quantification of low dose exposures.

Traditionally, the interpretation of dose–response relationships is based on models that take into account the modes of aberration formation and the biophysical processes of energy deposition. As an alternative, the nomenclature system PAINT suggests scoring colour junctions between painted and unpainted regions of structural chromosome changes without making any further assumptions. Whether this type of analysis (Tucker et al 1995b) is suitable for quantifying radiation-induced chromosome damage must be evaluated in the future.

Painting probes routinely cover about 10–22% of the total genomic DNA content. For a comparison of aberration frequencies measured with different chromosomes or chromosome combinations, with frequencies obtained from conventional chromosome analyses, partial-genome findings must be converted into whole-genome equivalents (Lucas et al 1992). This requires a DNA proportional distribution (i.e. according to their DNA content) of translocation break-points, an observation which is, however, not generally supported (Knehr et al 1994). Contradictory results also exist with respect to the ratio of symmetrical translocations to dicentrics. In theory, equal frequencies are expected; however, even with simultaneous centromere staining, radiation-induced translocation frequencies are found to be 1.5- to twofold higher than the frequencies of dicentrics. It was recently found that translocations in which the centromere belongs to an unpainted chromosome were present in excess, whereas those with a painted centromere occurred at the same frequency as dicentrics (Tucker et al 1995b).

Reliable long-term or retrospective biological dosimetry depends on the persistence of translocations with time post-exposure. Initial results on FISH translocation measurements obtained from single cases with accidental radiation exposure suggest a long-term stability (Straume et al 1992). A follow-up study of highly irradiated personnel at the Chernobyl reactor accident provided further evidence for the persistence of translocations: comparable dose estimates resulted from FISH analysis of stable translocations and conventional scoring of unstable dicentrics plus ring chromosomes, with the latter quantified by Q_{dr} (Salassidis et al 1994, 1995) (Figs 4 & 5). In addition, Giemsa banding revealed clonal aberrations in each case, and FISH revealed that target chromosomes were sometimes also involved. In the case of clonal expansion, a correction for a substantial contribution of clonal translocations to the total translocation frequency is mandatory for a reliable dose estimation.

Translocation yields in 19 Hiroshima atomic bomb survivors, examined some 45 years after exposure, compared well with those expected from an *in vitro* dose–response curve, although not a single clone has been reported (Lucas et al 1992). Contrary to these observations, Goiania data obtained in Leiden, suggest a decline of stable aberrations over the first few years after doses of more than 1 Gy (Natarajan et al 1997).

Because of the complex, largely unknown kinetics and variable individual dynamics of haematopoietic cell reproductive compartments — such as the bone marrow —

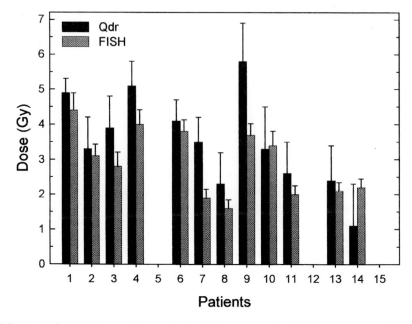

FIG. 4.   Individual dose estimates obtained from conventional chromosome analysis (Q_{dr} method) and translocation measurements by fluorescence *in situ* hybridization (FISH; painting of chromosomes 1, 4 and 12) from Chernobyl reactor personnel exposed during the accident. Error bars represent the upper 90% confidence interval. Patient numbers 5, 12 and 15 were members of liquidation teams arriving at the accident site a few days later.

further studies of various types of previous exposures are required for the validation of the long-term stability of translocations. It is also necessary to clarify whether dose-equivalent estimates obtained from translocation measurements many years after exposure can be related to the whole body or whether they are more representative of haemopoietic cell reproductive compartments. Cells containing unstable dicentrics are selected against during cell proliferation; therefore, preferentially undamaged cells or cells containing only transmissible symmetrical translocations (stable cells) will enter into the peripheral blood from these compartments. Assuming a temporal decline, both for unstable and stable aberrations through the natural attrition of T lymphocytes, with increasing time post-irradiation, a substantial fraction of damaged T lymphocytes should have been irradiated as stem cells or progenitor cells in the proliferating bone marrow, rather than as mature T lymphocytes in the peripheral blood. A differential radiosensitivity for these cell types could have some influence on the translocation frequency.

Due to the relatively high and variable background translocation frequencies, a large number of cells have to be analysed for the quantification of low level and chronic exposures by chromosome painting. For example, based on a control

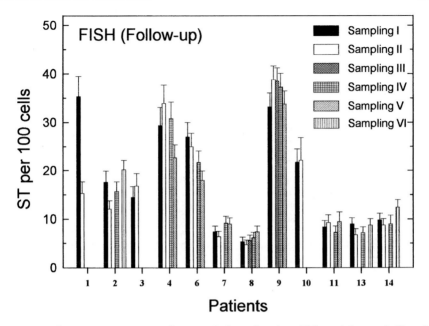

FIG. 5. Follow-up measurements of symmetrical translocations (ST) carried out at half-yearly intervals (I–VI) between September 1991 and July 1994 in the 12 highly exposed Chernobyl victims shown in Fig. 4. Excluding patient number 1, who is considered exceptional because the translocation frequencies at the two sampling times differ more than twofold, the temporal variation of the translocation frequencies was not statistically significant (multivariate χ^2 Poisson homogeneity test, $P > 0.05$; $\chi^2 = 43.5$; degrees of freedom = 31). FISH, fluorescence *in situ* hybridization. Error bars show S.E.M.

translocation frequency $F_p = 1.6 \times 10^{-3}$ in painted chromosomes 1, 4, 12 (full genome equivalent 5.1×10^{-3}), the detection of 300 mGy of γ-rays requires scoring a minimum of 4000 cells. This can be achieved routinely because FISH translocation analysis is about 10-fold quicker than conventional dicentric scoring. Automated metaphase detection and interactive translocation analysis will hopefully improve the situation further, so that this technique can be established as a retrospective biological dosemeter for practical application in radiation protection.

Acknowledgement

I thank H. Braselmann for mathematical–statistical treatment of the data and for preparation of the figures.

References

Bauchinger M 1995a Cytogenetic research after accidental radiation exposure. Stem Cells (suppl 1) 13:182–190

Bauchinger M 1995b Quantification of low-level radiation exposure by conventional chromosome aberration analysis. Mutat Res 339:177–189

Bauchinger M, Schmid E, Streng S, Dresp J 1983 Quantitative analysis of the chromosome damage at first division of human lymphocytes after ^{60}Co gamma-irradiation. Radiat Environ Biophys 22:225–229

Bauchinger M, Schmid E, Braselmann H, Willich N, Clemm C 1989 Time–effect relationship of chromosome aberrations in peripheral lymphocytes after radiation therapy for seminoma. Mutat Res 211:265–272

Bauchinger M, Schmid E, Zitzelsberger H, Braselmann H, Nahrstedt U 1993 Radiation-induced chromosome aberrations analyzed by 2-colour fluorescence in situ hybridization with composite whole chromosome-specific DNA probes and a pancentromeric DNA-probe. Int J Radiat Biol 64:179–184

Bender MA, Awa AA, Brooks AL et al 1988 Current status of cytogenetic procedures to detect and quantify previous exposures to radiation. Mutat Res 196:103–159

Bogen KT 1993 Reassessment of human peripheral T-lymphocyte lifespan deduced from cytogenetic and cytotoxic effects of radiation. Int J Radiat Biol 64:195–204

Buckton KE 1983 Chromosome aberrations in patients treated with X-irradiation for ankylosing spondylitis. In: Ishihara T, Sasaki MS (eds) Radiation-induced chromosome damage in man. Alan R. Liss, New York, p 491–511

Buckton KE, Hamilton GE, Paton L, Langlands AO 1978 Chromosome aberrations in irradiated ankylosing spondylitis patients. In: Evans HJ, Lloyd D (eds) Mutagen-induced chromosome damage in man. Yale University Press, London, p 142–150

Chadwick K, Gerber G (eds) 1991 Treatment and biological dosimetry of exposed persons: post-Chernobyl action. Unipub, Lanham, MD

Dolphin GW 1969 Biological dosimetry with particular reference to chromosome aberration analysis. A review of methods. In: Handling of radiation accidents: proceedings of a symposium organized in collaboration with WHO in Vienna, 1969. International Atomic Energy Agency, Vienna, p 215–224

Griffin CS, Marsden SJ, Stevens DL Simpson P, Savage JRK 1995 Frequencies of complex chromosome exchange aberrations induced by Pu-238 alpha-particles and detected by fluorescence in situ hybridization using single chromosome-specific probes. Int J Radiat Biol 67:431–439

IAEA 1986a Summary report on post-accident. Review meeting on the Chernobyl accident. International Atomic Energy Agency, Vienna

IAEA 1986b Biological dosimetry. Chromosomal aberration analysis for dose assessment. International Atomic Energy Agency, Vienna

IAEA 1988 A report on the Goiania (Brazil) radiation accident. International Atomic Energy Agency, Vienna

Knehr S, Zitzelsberger H, Braselmann H, Bauchinger M 1994 Analysis for DNA-proportional distribution of radiation-induced chromosome aberrations in various triple combinations of human chromosomes using fluorescence in situ hybridization. Int J Radiat Biol 65:683–690

Kulka U, Huber R, Müller P, Knehr S, Bauchinger M 1995 Combined FISH painting and harlequin staining for cell cycle-controlled chromosme analysis in human lymphocytes. Int J Radiat Biol 68:25–27

Léonard A, Deknudt GH, Léonard ED 1988 Persistence of chromosome aberrations in an accidentally irradiated subject. Radiat Prot Dosimetry 22:55–57

Littlefield LG, Joiner EE, Colyer SP, Ricks RC, Lushbaugh CC, Hutada-Monroy R 1991 The 1989 San Salvador ^{60}Co radiation accident: cytogenetic dosimetry and follow-up evaluations in three accident victims. Radiat Prot Dosimetry 35:115–123

Lucas JN, Awa A, Straume T et al 1992 Rapid translocation frequency analysis in humans decades after exposure to ionizing radiation. Int J Radiat Biol 62:53–63

Natarajan AT, Darroudi F, Hadjidekova V et al 1997 Biological dosimetric studies in Goiania accident. In: Scientific bases for decision making after a radioactive contamination of an urban environment. International Atomic Energy Agency, Vienna, in press

Pinkel D, Straume T, Gray JW 1986 Cytogenetic analysis using high-sensitivity fluorescence hybridization. Proc Natl Acad Sci USA 83:2934–2938

Ramalho AT, Nascimento RCH, Natarajan AT 1988 Dose assessments by cytogenetic analysis in the Goiania (Brazil) radiation accident. Radiat Prot Dosimetry 25:97–100

Salassidis K, Schmid E, Peter RU, Braselmann H, Bauchinger M 1994 Dicentric and translocation analysis for retrospective dose estimation in humans exposed to ionising radiation during the Chernobyl nuclear power plant accident. Mutat Res 311:39–48

Salassidis K, Georgiadou-Schumacher V, Braselmann H, Müller P, Peter RU, Bauchinger M 1995 Chromosome painting in highly irradiated Chernobyl victims: a follow-up study to evaluate the stability of symmetrical translocations and the influence of clonal aberrations for retrospective dose estimation. Int J Radiat Biol 68:257–262

Sasaki MS 1983 Use of lymphocyte chromosome aberrations in biological dosimetry: possibilities an limitations. In: Ishihara T, Sasaki MS (eds) Radiation-induced chromosome damage in man. Alan R. Liss, New York, p 585–604

Savage JRK, Simpson PJ 1994 FISH 'painting' patterns resulting from complex exchanges. Mutat Res 312:51–60

Simpson PJ, Savage JRK 1994 Identification of X-ray-induced complex chromosome exchanges using fluorescence *in situ* hybridization: a comparison at 2 doses. Int J Radiat Biol 66:629–632

Simpson PJ, Savage JRK 1995 Estimating the true frequency of X-ray-induced complex chromosome exchanges using fluorescence *in situ* hybridisation. Int J Radiat Biol 67:37–45

Straume T, Lucas JD, Tucker WL, Bigbee AT, Langlois RG 1992 Biodosimetry for a radiation worker using multiple assays. Health Phys 62:122–130

Trepel F 1975 Kinetik lymphatischer Zellen. In: Theml H, Begemann H (eds) Lymphozyt und klinische Immunologie. Springer-Verlag, Berlin, p 16–26

Trepel F 1976 Das lymphatische Zellsystem: Struktur, allgemeine Physiologie und allgemeine Pathophysiologie. In: Begemann H (ed) Blut und Blutkrankheiten, Teil 3, Leukozytäres und retikuläres System I. Springer-Verlag, Berlin, p 1–191

Tucker JD, Morgan WF, Awa AA et al 1995a A proposed system for scoring structural aberrations detected by chromosome painting. Cytogenet Cell Genet 68:211–221

Tucker JD, Lee DA, Moore DH 1995b Validation of chromosome painting. 2. A detailed analysis of aberrations following high doses of ionizing radiation *in vitro*. Int J Radiat Biol 67:19–28

Weier H-UG, Lucas, JN, Poggensee M, Segraves R, Pinkel D, Gray JW 1991 Two-color hybridization with high complexity chromosome-specific probes and a degenerate alpha satellite probe DNA allows unambiguous discrimination between symmetrical and asymmetrical translocations. Chromosoma 100:311–317

DISCUSSION

Goldman: You performed several different repeat estimates. Were these repeats performed on the same person or on different people?

Bauchinger: On the same person. We had 12 individuals and we tried to obtain several samples from each individual. Unfortunately, in some cases we could only obtain two, but for others we obtained up to six samples.

Balonov: What is the normal half-life of the chromosome aberrations in lymphocytes?

Bauchinger: Depending on the model that we use, it takes about 3–3.5 years for dicentrics to disappear from the circulating blood. Bogen (1993) has developed a new approach, using a two-compartment model which postulates that two major T lymphocyte subpopulations—one short-lived, one long-lived—may be better suited to this situation. Our data on the temporal decline of unstable aberrations in patients therapeutically irradiated for seminoma could be described by a time–hyperbolic model (Bauchinger et al 1989), i.e. immediately and 1720 days after radiation therapy half-lives of 0.4 and 3.6 years, respectively, were estimated. For the 15 subjects exposed during the 1987 Goiania accident in Brazil, a two-phase exponential function has been postulated for the disappearance of unstable aberrations: for exposures above 1 Gy, the average half-time for elimination of dicentrics and rings was 110 days post-exposure and for exposures below 1 Gy it was 160 days post-exposure (Ramalho et al 1995).

Streffer: I am worried by the large interindividual differences between the 15 people analysed after the Goiania accident. Can you explain this?

Bauchinger: No, I can't, I've discussed this problem with A. T. Natarajan (MGC, Department of Radiation Genetics and Chemical Mutagenesis, State University of Leiden, The Netherlands). It is possible that different T lymphocyte populations are involved. What surprises me is that the development of clonal aberrations has not been observed in either the 15 Goiania cases (Straume et al 1991) or the 20 Hiroshima atomic bomb survivors (Lucas et al 1992) examined by fluorescence *in situ* hybridization (FISH) analysis. So far, we have defined two expanding clones in our highly irradiated Chernobyl cases and we have strong evidence for even more. This is what one should expect, because with increasing time post-exposure, stem cell or progenitor cells carrying stable chromosomal aberrations that do not interfere with normal mitotic divisions should be able to generate a substantial number of clonal cells.

Paretzke: How do you identify them as being clones? Is it possible that other researchers have overlooked them?

Bauchinger: In principle, there is a danger of overlooking the clones if one only does conventional scoring. For example, the translocation t(1q25;13q14) in one of our Chernobyl cases cannot be detected by conventional scoring, and FISH analysis alone does not guarantee that it is a clonal aberration. If a certain target chromosome is frequently involved in stable translocations this can give a strong indication for the existence of a clone. For a conclusive evaluation, G-banding is also required to define the identical breakpoints.

Whicker: Has the FISH technique been applied to species other than humans?

Bauchinger: Results have been published for the mouse (Breneman et al 1993, Boei et al 1994) and whole-chromosome probes have also recently become available for the Chinese hamster (Balajee et al 1995). In principle, it can be applied to any species, as long as the right probes are available.

Whicker: I have been working on some reservoirs at the Savannah River site, which have been contaminated with radiocaesium and radiostrontium for 30 years. Turtles live in these reservoirs, and we have not detected any obvious abnormalities in these turtles. It would be interesting to use the FISH technique to determine whether chromosomal changes are present that have accumulated over a long period of time. They are being exposed to up to 0.01 Gy/day in certain habitats, so over a period of several years they're getting reasonable doses.

Bauchinger: You would have to select specific chromosomes for the analysis. This involves, for example, microdissection of these chromosomes and repressing hybridization of other chromosomes once you have made your probe. Obtaining specific probes in this way is not an easy task.

Streffer: We are using this technique in our laboratory for mice because probes for all the murine chromosomes are now available commercially. Have you any idea if the persistence of the effect is dependent on the dose? Within a dose range where there are chromosomal aberrations in virtually every T lymphocyte, one would expect that there would also be extensive cell loss. There may also be a fading of the signal, as was observed for the dicentrics.

Bauchinger: There is a dose dependence for chromosomal aberrations in various groups of radiation-exposed persons but the persistence is less clear. With increasing time after exposure, the frequencies of both unstable and stable cells should be reduced in the peripheral blood. If we assume a repopulation from the haematopoietic centres, only cells without aberrations or those carrying stable translocations should be capable of proliferation. The reconstituted cell population should express the identical aberration, i.e. it is of clonal origin. Therefore, the probability of finding clones should increase with time after exposure. This creates the problem of whether the biological dose estimate derived from stable chromosome aberration frequencies is still representative for an equivalent whole-body dose or whether it must be related only to the haematopoietic stem cell or the progenitor pool. We don't have enough data to resolve this yet.

Paretzke: Could this problem be solved by analysing blood of partially irradiated patients undergoing cancer radiotherapy? Their bone marrow could have been exposed to a known therapeutic dose, and one could calculate the dose to other parts of the body.

Bauchinger: We have thought of such an approach but we are currently planning an examination first to calibrate our system. We would like to have some exact dose exposure information on, for example, nuclear power plant workers because although we know the occupational doses they have received for more than 20 or 30 years, we have still insufficient information on the long-term stability of symmetrical translocations, and therefore on the problem of whether painting analysis is a suitable means for integrating biodosimetry. If we obtain these, we should be able to compare their accumulated physical doses with those obtained from translocation measurements, so that we can calculate the efficiency.

Goldman: If you did the dosimetry on internally exposed Russian Techa river inhabitants, whose exposure was predominantly from the yttrium and strontium beta particles in the bone marrow (but not anywhere else), you would have the opportunity to look at a set of stem cells as opposed to whole-body irradiation. You would also have a unique opportunity to see the accumulation of stable aberrations and the decrease in the unstable ones. The ratios would be different in these people. Have you looked at this?

Bauchinger: Yes. We have an ongoing programme where we plan to examine 100 highly exposed radiation workers of the former Soviet Union nuclear industrial production company Mayak and 100 Techa riverside residents exposed to radioactive liquid discharge of Mayak in the area of the Southern Urals in the 1950s. So far we have done about 50 of each. For the Mayak data, we have cells with complex chromosome aberrations and so far we have observed a threefold increased frequency of symmetrical translocations compared to controls. We didn't see such an increase for the Techa riverside population.

Paretzke: If you knew the physical dose, would a chromosome analysis of a person be sufficient to determine whether they were prone to develop leukaemia or not?

Bauchinger: It is possible, but it would require a different approach. We are currently looking at specific stable chromosomes using painting probes. It is possible to use DNA probes for specific genes or oncogenes. If you know that there is a translocation process which is indicative of a particular marker chromosome, for example the Philadelphia chromosome t(9;22), then you can use specific locus probes to detect this marker in interphase cells. This is what we have done. We first looked at a few metaphase preparations to check the probes were working and then we analysed hundreds of cells in interphase. In four cases we observed an increased frequency of the translocation that juxtaposes the proto-oncogene ABL on chromosome 9 with the BCR gene on chromosome 22. Although the BCR/ABL rearrangement is a typical molecular event in chronic myeloid leukaemia, we don't know yet whether in the present cases it is an early sign of oncogenicity.

Paretzke: Unfortunately, at present we don't know many tumours that are associated with specific chromosomal aberrations. This number of tumours may increase with our increasing understanding of molecular biology. This may be an excellent biological way of identifying people at risk of developing a tumour, irrespective of their physical radiation dose.

Bauchinger: It may also be a means of detecting radiospecific changes at the chromosome and DNA level.

Paretzke: Could you mention some of the cytogenetic analyses that you have done on cells from thyroid tumours obtained from children in Belarus and from children who have had radiation therapy for thyroid cancer in Munich?

Bauchinger: These are preliminary results. So far, we have no evidence for a radiospecific change, i.e. there is no specific chromosomal marker for thyroid tumours. However, when these are compared to cases who underwent therapeutic irradiation with very high doses, there were some cases that had a similar amount of symmetrical translocations. In a large number of cases we didn't see anything. Therefore, the differential exposure of the children seems to be critical.

Streffer: We are also doing some studies on thyroid carcinomas, and we have been looking for mutations in the p53 gene. We also had the idea that specific changes which occur after irradiation may be useful for identifying whether a particular individual tumour has a higher probability of being caused by irradiation than by other causes. I think it is possible to do this but we have been disappointed with the results of our own studies. The p53 gene is often mutated in human tumours, but the frequency of such mutations in thyroid carcinomas is comparatively low. We have studied exons 1–11 in 70 tumours, and we have only found 10 mutations, most of which occur in exons 6 and 7. Therefore, it seems that there is no relationship between these mutations and the development of a tumour.

Bauchinger: We have similar results. We have looked at 60 thyroid tumour samples (29 childhood tumours from Belarus and 31 from juveniles and adults without radiation history for control). In the reference group, seven different mutations in the p53 gene were found on exons 5 to 8 but none were observed among the nine papillary carcinomas. The three mutations found in the 22 papillary type carcinomas of the Belarussian cases were concentrated only in codon 213 of exon 6, which is rather peculiar.

Streffer: I would like to mention another cytogenetic technique, namely the micronucleus technique, which is performed on both T and B lymphocytes. The specificity with respect to ionizing radiation is less than for the dicentric aberrations because micronuclei are not only produced by ionizing irradiation but also by a number of chemicals. On the other hand, it can be used as a screening procedure for environmental pollution. One of the problems with the technique is the persistence of the effect, i.e. in a similar fashion to the dicentrics, it fades after some months or years. The sensitivity, at least in our hands, is in the range of 0.2–0.5 Gy, depending on which cells we are analysing. In B lymphocytes we can detect a dose of about 0.2 Gy; however, there are some experimental difficulties involving the isolation of B lymphocytes that we have to consider. The maximum dose is in the range of 3–5 Gy. Therefore, it is used for a similar dose range as the dicentric analysis, although the lower limit may be a little less than the dicentric analysis. We also have results from our laboratory (Müller et al 1995) on external and internal irradiation, LET dependence and dose rate dependence. All these results are comparable to those for the dicentric analysis. However, there are some advantages of this technique over the dicentric analysis. It is much easier and quicker to do, and therefore a larger number of samples can be analysed. The process can also be fully automated, so there is a high level of reproducibility and it can be performed all day and all night. Consequently, it is a useful technique, especially if large numbers of people, for example those exposed as a result of an accident, have to be analysed.

References

Balajee AS, Dominguez I, Natarajan AT 1995 Construction of Chinese hamster-specific DNA libraries and their use in the analysis of spontaneous chromosome rearrangements in different cell lines. Cytogenet Cell Genet 70:95–101

Bauchinger M, Schmid E, Braselmann H, Willich N, Clemm C 1989 Time–effect relationship of chromosome aberrations in peripheral lymphocytes after radiation therapy for seminoma. Mutat Res 211:265–272

Boei JJWA, Balajee AS, De Boer P, Aten JA, Mullenders LHF, Natarajan AT 1994 Construction of mouse chromosome-specific DNA libraries and their use for the detection of X-ray-induced aberrations. Int J Radiat Biol 65:583–590

Bogen KT 1993 Reassessment of human peripheral T-lymphocyte lifespan deduced from cytogenetic and cytotoxic effects of radiation. Int J Radiat Biol 64:195–204

Breneman JW, Ramsey MJ, Lee DA, Eveleth GG, Minkler JL, Tucker JD 1993 The development of chromosome-specific composite DNA probes for the mouse and their application to chromosome painting. Chromosoma 102:591–598

Müller W-U, Streffer C, Wuttke K 1995 Micronucleus determination as a means to assess radiation exposure. Stem Cells 13:199–206

Ramalho AT, Curado MP, Natarajan AT 1995 Lifespan of human lymphocytes estimated during a six year cytogenetic follow-up of individuals accidentally exposed in the 1987 radiological accident in Brazil. Mutation Res 331:47–54

Straume T, Lucas JD, Tucker WL, Bigbee AT, Langlois RG 1992 Biodosimetry for a radiation worker using multiple assays. Health Phys 62:122–130

Mental health, stress and risk perception: insights from psychological research

Ortwin Renn

Center of Technology Assessment, Industriestrasse 5, D-70565 Stuttgart, Germany

Abstract. Risk perceptions are only slightly correlated with the expected values of a probability distribution for negative health impacts. Psychometric studies have documented that context variables such as dread or personal control are important predictors for the perceived seriousness of risk. Studies about cultural patterns of risk perceptions emphasize different response sets to risk information, depending on cultural priorities such as social justice versus personal freedom. This chapter reports the major psychological research results pertaining to the factors that govern individual risk perception and discusses the psychometric effects due to people's risk perception and the experience of severe stress. The relative importance of the psychometric context variables, the signals pertaining to each health risks and symbolic beliefs are explained.

1997 Health impacts of large releases of radionuclides. Wiley, Chichester (Ciba Foundation Symposium 203) p 205–231

The beginning of risk analysis was marked by technical analyses of calculating probabilities for undesirable outcomes of human activities or natural events based on observed frequencies of these outcomes in the past. Technical analysis provides society with a narrow definition of undesirable effects and confines possibilities to numerical probabilities based on relative frequencies. For example, many health physicists have calculated the probability of developing cancer as a function of radioactive intake. Based on animal studies or epidemiological research, dose–response functions are constructed that model the likelihood of an individual to be affected by the respective health disease depending on the dose of the disease-causing agent. Disease is then conceptualized as a chemical or bio-kinetic reaction to an external stimulus. Psychosomatic effects are often neglected when risk is conceptualized in such a way. However, this narrowness is a virtue as much as it is a shortcoming. Focused on 'real' health effects or ecological damage, technical analyses are based on a societal consensus of undesirability and a (positivistic) methodology that assures equal treatment for all risks under consideration. The price we pay for this methodological rigour is the simplicity of an abstraction we make from the culture and context of risk-taking behaviour.

The social science perspectives on risk broaden the scope of undesirable effects, include other ways to express possibilities and likelihood, and expand the understanding of reality to include the interpretations of undesirable events and 'socially constructed' realities, including perceptions and psychosomatic impacts (Renn 1992). It seems advisable to conceptualize risk partly as a social construct and partly as an objective property of a hazard or event (Renn 1992, Renn et al 1992, cf. Short 1989). To treat risk as both an objective property and a social construct avoids the problem of total relativism on the one hand and of technological determinism on the other hand. Manifestations of risk, i.e. accidents or releases of harmful substances or radionuclides, are called 'hazardous events'. These events are real and objective — in the sense that people or the environment are harmed. Hazardous events remain largely irrelevant in the social context unless they are observed by humans and communicated to others (Luhmann 1986). Perceptions of risk, i.e. the social and individual processing of risk-related signals (physical and communicative) lead to somatic responses and social actions. The experience of risk is therefore not only an experience of physical harm but the result of a process by which individuals or groups learn to acquire or create interpretations of hazards. These interpretations provide rules of how to select, order, and often explain, signals from the physical world.

This chapter attempts to review the present knowledge of risk perception and to explain the psychological and social factors that shape the experience of risk. The main objective of this chapter is to integrate the results of psychological, sociological and medical studies, and present the major findings of the social sciences as they seem relevant for risk perception and stress inducement.

How do people perceive risks?

Attention and selection filters

Today's society provides an abundance of information, much more than any individual can digest. It is assumed that the average person is exposed to 7000 bits of information each day of which s/he perceives around 700, acknowledges 70, stores seven in the short-term memory and may remember less than one in the longer term. Most information to which the average person is exposed will be ignored. This is not a malicious act but a sheer necessity in order to reduce the amount of information a person can process in a given time.

The attention and selection process is not random, although random elements may play a role. People have developed special strategies to select information that they feel is relevant to them. This is also true for risk information. The major criteria for selection are ability and motivation (Chaiken & Stangor 1987). Ability refers to the physical possibility that the receiver can follow the message without distraction, and

TABLE 1   **Conditions and requirements for information selection**

Conditions	Elements of Conditions
Ability	Physical access to information
	Time to process information
	Absence of sources of distraction
Motivation	Reference to personal interests, salient values or self-esteem
	Inducement of personal involvement with issue, the content or the source

motivation to the readiness and interest of the receiver to process the message. The conditions for both ability and motivation are listed in Table 1.

Three conditions have to be met to satisfy the criterion of ability: the information has to be accessible; the receiver must have the time to process the information; and other sources of distraction should be absent. Several factors influence the motivation of a receiver to process the information actively. The information content has to be relevant (referring to personal interests, salient values or self-esteem) and it should trigger personal involvement (with the issue, the content or the source). Both motivational factors are reinforced if the receiver has some prior knowledge or interest in the subject or is in need for new arguments to back up his/her point of view. If both criteria are met, the individual selects the information. However, to economize further on time, s/he is going to evaluate whether it is necessary to study the content of the information in detail or to make a fast judgement according to some salient cues in the message received. The first strategy refers to the central route of information processing, and the second to the peripheral route (Petty & Cacioppo 1986, Renn & Levine 1991). The central route is taken when the receiver is so highly motivated by the message that s/he studies each argument carefully. The peripheral route is taken when the receiver is less inclined to deal with each argument, but forms an opinion or even an attitude on the basis of simple cues and heuristics (Figs 1 & 2).

The major difference between the peripheral and central routes lies in the process of the evaluation of the message. In the central mode, the receiver performs two types of evaluation: first, an assessment of th e probability that each argument is true; and second, an assignment of weight to each argument according to the personal salience of the argument's content. The credibility of each argument can be tested by referring to personal experience, plausibility and perceived motives of the communicator. The major incentives for changing an attitude in the central mode are the proximity with and the affinity to one's own interests, values and world views. In the peripheral mode, receivers do not bother to deal with each argument separately, but look for easily accessible clues to make their judgement on the whole package. Examples of such cues are the length of a message, the number of arguments, the package (e.g. colour,

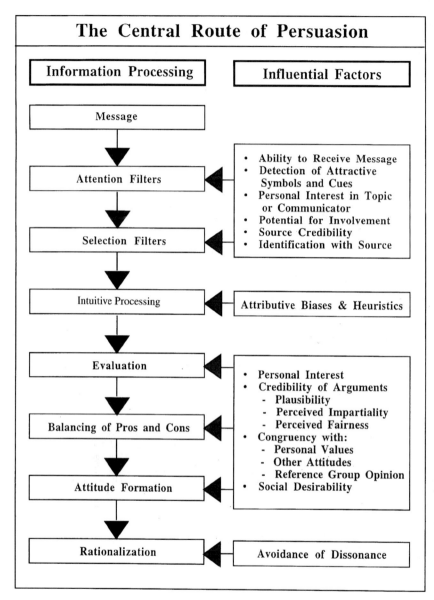

FIG. 1.   The central route of information processing. In the central mode the receiver performs two types of evaluations: (1) an assessment of the probability that each argument is true; (2) an assignment of weight to each argument according to the personal salience of the argument's content. The major incentives for changing an attitude in the central mode are the proximity with and the affinity to one's own interests, values and world views.

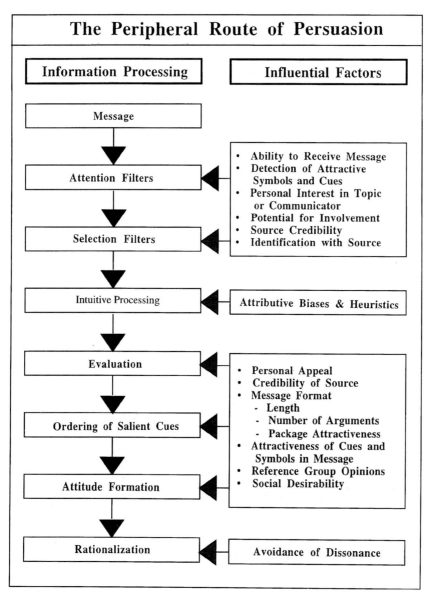

FIG. 2. The peripheral route of information processing. In the peripheral mode, receivers do not bother to deal with each argument separately but look for easily accessible clues to make their judgement on the whole package. Examples, of such cues are the length of a message, the number of arguments, the package (e.g. colour, paper and graphic appeal) and the presence of symbolic signals that trigger immediate emotional responses.

paper and graphic appeal) and the presence of symbolic signals that trigger immediate emotional responses (cf. Kasperson et al 1988).

The difference between the central and the peripheral route can be illustrated by drawing on the experiences from the perception of nuclear energy. Many people feel that energy is such an important commodity for their life that they study all the information on potential impacts and threats in order to understand the issues and trade-offs involved. Others base their judgements on cues such as behaviour of neighbours (do they worry about the nearby nuclear power plant?) or sporadic news reports about nuclear problems. Communicating with the first group demands thorough argumentation and detailed analysis of decision options (which usually deters the peripherally interested persons); communicating with the second group requires the use of entertaining and appealing cues such as coloured brochures and trust-building public relations (which unfortunately alienate the centrally interested group). A good risk communicator should try to identify the type of audience (central or peripheral) before designing the communication process.

Intuitive heuristics

Once information has been received, common-sense mechanisms process the information and help the receiver to draw inferences. These processes are called intuitive heuristics. They are particularly important for risk perception because they relate to the mechanisms of processing probabilistic information. Early psychological studies focused on personal preferences for probabilities and attempted to explain why individuals do not base their risk judgements on expected values, i.e. the product of probability and magnitude of an adverse effect (Pollatsek & Tversky 1970, Lopes 1983). One of the interesting results of these investigations was the discovery of systematic patterns of probabilistic reasoning that are well suited for most everyday situations. People are risk averse if the stakes of losses are high and risk prone if the stakes for gains are high (Kahneman & Tversky 1979). Furthermore, many people balance their risk taking behaviour by pursuing an optimal risk strategy, which does not maximize their benefits but assures both a satisfactory pay-off and the avoidance of major disasters (Luce & Weber 1986).

One example of such a strategy is to use the mini–max rule for making decisions. This rule implies that people try to minimize post-decisional regret by choosing the option that has the least potential for a disaster regardless of probabilities. Many energy managers have difficulties in understanding why a facility such as coal-fired power station, with a fairly large concentration of pollutants that may cause chronic effects but hardly any fatalities, is less feared by many people than a minute amount of a radioactive material that has the potential to cause cancer, but in its present concentration is far below the threshold of causing harm to public health. The answer, of course, is that people often use the mini–max rule for judging risks and are thus more afraid of a potentially toxic material (regardless of concentration) than of a more common but less harmful pollutant. The use of this rule is not irrational (Lee

TABLE 2   Intuitive biases of risk perception

Biases	Description
Availability	Events that come to people's mind are immediately rated as more probable than events that are less mentally available
Anchoring effect	Probabilities are adjusted to the information available or the perceived significance of the information
Representativeness	Singular events experienced in person or associated with properties of an event are regarded as more typical than information based on frequencies
Avoidance of cognitive dissonance	Information that challenges perceived probabilities that are already part of a belief system will either be ignored or down-played

1981). It has evolved over a long evolution of human behaviour as a fairly successful strategy to cope with uncertainty (better safe than sorry).

Second, more specific studies on the perception of probabilities in decision making identified several biases in people's ability to draw inferences from probabilistic information (Festinger 1957, Kahneman & Tversky 1979, Ross 1977). These biases are summarized in Table 2.

Risk managers and public health professionals should be aware of these biases because they are found in public perception and may be one of the underlying causes for the observed public response. For example, the frequent media coverage about leukaemia cases based on exposure to radioactive substances has alarmed the public and promoted a response of outrage based on the availability bias.

Semantic images

Psychological research has revealed different meanings of risk depending on the context in which the term is used. In the technical sciences the term risk denotes the probability of adverse effects, whereas the everyday use of the term risk has different connotations. Table 3 illustrates the main semantic images with respect to technological risk (Renn 1984, 1989).

Risk as a pending danger (Damocles' sword).   Risks are seen as a random threat that can trigger a disaster without prior notice and without sufficient time to cope with the hazard involved. This image is linked to artificial risk sources with large catastrophic potential. The magnitude of the probability is not considered. It is rather the randomness itself that evokes fear and avoidance responses. Natural disasters, in contrast, are perceived as regularly occurring and thus predictable or related to a special pattern of occurrence (causal, temporal or magic). The image of pending

TABLE 3   The four semantic images of risk in public perception

Semantic image	Attributes
Pending danger (Damocles' sword)	Artificial risk source
	Large catastrophic potential
	Inequitable risk–benefit distribution
	Perception of randomness as a threat
Slow killers (Pandora's box)	(Artificial) Ingredient in food, water, or air
	Delayed effects; non-catastrophic
	Contingent on information rather than experience
	Quest for deterministic risk management
	Strong incentive for blame
Cost–benefit ratio (Athena's scale)	Confined to monetary gains and losses
	Orientation towards variance of distribution rather than expected value
	Asymmetry between risks and gains
	Dominance of probabilistic thinking
Avocational thrill (Hercules' image)	Personal control over degree of risk
	Personal skills necessary to master danger
	Voluntary activity
	Non-catastrophic consequences

danger is therefore particularly prevalent in the perception of large-scale technologies. Nuclear power plants are a prime example of this semantic category.

Slow killers (Pandora's box).   Risk is seen as an invisible threat to one's health or well-being. Effects are usually delayed and affect only few people at the same time. Knowledge about these risks is based on information by others rather than on personal experience. These risks pose a major demand for trustworthiness in those institutions that provide information and manage the hazard. If trust is lost, people demand immediate actions and assign blame to these institutions even if the risks are small. Typical examples of this risk class are food additives, pesticides and radioactive substances. Due to the importance of trust in monitoring and managing slow killers, nuclear risk managers should place a major effort to improve their trustworthiness and credibility in the community. Later in this chapter, some recommendations to reach this goal will be made.

Cost–benefit ratio (Athena's scale).   Risks are perceived as a balancing of gains and losses. This concept of risk comes closest to the technical understanding of risk. However, this image is only used in peoples' perceptions of monetary gains and losses. Typical examples are betting and gambling, both of which require sophisticated probabilistic reasoning. People are normally able to perform such probabilistic reasoning but only in the context of gambling, lotteries, financial investment and insurance. Laboratory experiments show that people orient their judgement about lotteries more towards the variance of losses and gains than towards the expected value (Pollatsek & Tversky 1970).

Avocational thrill (Hercules' theme). Often risks are actively explored and desired (Machlis & Rosa 1990). These risks include all activities for which personal skills are necessary to master the dangerous situation. The thrill is derived from the enjoyment of having control over one's environment or oneself. Such risks are always voluntary and allow personal control over the degree of riskiness.

Qualitative risk characteristics

In addition to the images that are linked to different risk contexts, the type of risk involved and its situational characteristics shape individual risk estimations and evaluations (Slovic 1987, Renn 1990a,b). Psychometric methods have been employed to explore these qualitative characteristics of risks. The following contextual variables of risk have been found to affect the perceived seriousness of risks (Slovic et al 1981, Vlek & Stallen 1981, Renn 1986, 1990a,b, Covello 1983, Gould et al 1988).

The expected number of fatalities or losses. Although the perceived average number of fatalities correlates with the perceived riskiness of a technology or activity, the relationship is weak and generally explains less than 20% of the declared variance. The major disagreement between technical risk analysis and risk perception is not on the number of affected persons, but on the importance of this information for evaluating the seriousness of risk.

The catastrophic potential. Most people show distinctive preferences among choices with identical expected values (average risk). Low probability, high consequence risks are usually perceived as more threatening than more probable risks with low or medium consequences. This preference for low consequence risk is another expression of the application of the mini–max rule.

Situational characteristics. Surveys and experiments have revealed that perception of risks is influenced by a series of perceived properties of the risk source or the risk situation. These properties are called qualitative characteristics. Table 4 lists the major qualitative characteristics and their influence on risk perception. In addition to these qualitative factors, equity issues play a major role in risk perception. The more risks are seen as unfair for the exposed population, the more they are judged as severe and unacceptable (Kasperson & Kasperson 1983, Short 1984). The perception of nuclear health risks is usually linked to an absence of personal control and the preponderance of dread thus amplifying the impression of seriousness.

TABLE 4   List of important qualitative risk characteristics

Qualitative characteristics	_Direction of influence_
Personal control	Increases risk tolerance
Institutional control	Depends on confidence in institutional perform
Voluntariness	Increases risk tolerance
Familiarity	Increases tisk tolerance
Dread	Decreases risk tolerance
Inequitable distribution of risks and benefits	Depends on individual utility, strong social incentive for rejecting risks
Artificiality of risk source	Amplifies attention to risk, often decreases risk tolerance
Blame	Increases quest for social and political responses

The beliefs associated with the cause of risk.   The perception of risk is often part of an attitude that a person holds about the cause of the risk, i.e. a technology, human activity or natural event. Attitudes encompass a series of beliefs about the nature, consequences, history and justifiability of a risk cause (Thomas et al 1980, Otway & Thomas 1982). Due to the tendency to avoid cognitive dissonance, i.e. emotional stress caused by conflicting beliefs (Festinger 1957), most people are inclined to perceive risks as more serious and threatening if the other beliefs contain negative connotations and vice versa. A person who believes that the energy industry is guided by greed and profit is more likely to think that the risks of nuclear power are only the 'tip of an iceberg'. On the other hand, a person who believes that energy utilities are fair players with a desired good and needed services is likely to link routine releases of small amounts of radioactive substances with unpleasant, but essentially manageable, by-products of energy generation. Often risk perception is a product of these underlying beliefs rather than the cause of these beliefs (Clarke 1989).

It should be noted that the estimation of seriousness and the judgement about acceptability are closely related in risk perception. The analytical separation in risk estimation, evaluation and management, as exercised by most technical risk experts (NRC 1983), is not paralleled in public perception. Most people integrate information about the magnitude of the risk, the fairness of the risk situation and other qualitative factors into their overall judgement about the (perceived) seriousness of the respective risk.

Public responses to risk

Role and functions of the media in shaping risk perception

All mechanisms of perception are contingent on information derived from either personal experience, interaction with others or intermediary sources. A vast amount of information about risks stems from intermediary sources. People develop attitudes and positions with respect to risky technologies and or activities on the basis of second-hand information. This information is transmitted by the media. Many beliefs about risks and risk sources are hence shaped, or at least influenced, by the information and evaluations that the media transmit to their consumers. The media perform a dual role in the communication process: first, they collect information from primary sources and process this information by applying professional and institutional rules that govern the selection of received messages and their interpretation; and second, they send information to the final receiver.

The transformation process of messages during transmission has been a popular topic of communication research. From a theoretical point of view, many different concepts about the nature of this transformation have been suggested in the literature (Peters 1984, 1991, Peltu 1985, Lee 1986). The basic differences between these approaches may be confined to two major questions. Are the media creating new messages or are they reflecting existing messages? How biased are journalists in their coverage *vis-à-vis* their own social convictions and external pressures? Both questions have yet to be answered (Peltu 1985, Lichtenberg & MacLean 1988).

With respect to the first question, the literature suggested a strong influence of the media on public opinion in the early years of communication research. Through extensive testing, however, this hypothesis was later substituted by the hypothesis that the media set the agenda, but do not change the attitudes or the values of the audience with respect to the issues on the agenda (McCombs & Shaw 1972, Peltu 1985, Lichtenberg & MacLean 1988). Only in the long term have the media a lasting effect on the attitude and value structure of their consumers.

With respect to the second question, evidence has been gathered to support almost all possible viewpoints. Political and commercial pressures have been detected in media coverage as well as courageous news reports in conflict with all vested interests. Cultural biases within the journalistic community have been found, but also a variety of different political and social attitudes exist among journalists. In short: the extremes that media are mere reflectors of reality or that they are docile instruments of social pressure groups may occasionally be true, but they are not the rule. In reality, the situation is more complex: media coverage is neither dependent on external pressures nor an autonomous subsystem within society (Raymond 1985). It reflects internalized individual values, organizational rules and external expectations. It depends on the issue itself, the institutional context and the political salience of the issue which, of these three factors, is likely to dominate the transformation process. A universal theory of how this transformation takes place is therefore not likely to evolve. Some of the common characteristics of media coverage deserve some attention, however.

(1)   The media construct reality, and the readers construct their understanding of the media report (Dunwoody 1992). These constructions are the results of mental and professional frames that journalists use in selecting and recoding information. Construction does not imply that the coverage is independent of

the real events, but there is ample evidence that the media amplify some elements and down-play others when processing information (Wilkins & Patterson 1987, Sood et al 1987). For example, the number of fatalities is a rather weak indicator for the amount of coverage in risk issues, whereas the degree of social conflict arising from a risk debate correlates high with media coverage (Adams 1986).

(2) The media direct their attention to events, not continuous developments. An accident-free performance of a technology over many years is not newsworthy, unless it is framed as an event (such as a public celebration). Likewise, slow changes of the climate become hot news issues only if they can be linked to a conference, an exceptionally hot summer (such as 1988 in the USA) or political statements (Peltu 1988).

(3) The media have no internal mechanism to resolve conflicts among experts. Journalists have neither the time nor the qualification to find out who is right in a scientific debate. The most frequently used method to handle competing scientific evidence in the media is to give each side room to state or justify claims (Peters 1991). Most journalists have lists of people who will provide counter-statements to any statement that they encounter when working on a story. Neither quality of evidence nor proportionality (with respect to number of dissidents or professional qualification) determine the amount of coverage. The amount is either equally distributed among camps, or biased towards the preferences of the journalist or towards the editorial style of the respective medium. The media in a pluralistic society tend to reinforce diversity, dissent and relativity of values (Rubin 1987).

Institutional trust and confidence

As personal experience of risk has been replaced by information about risks and individual control over risk by institutional risk management, trust in institutional performance has been the major key for risk responses. Trust in control institutions is able to compensate for a negative perception, and distrust may lead people to oppose risks even when they are perceived as small. Trust can be substructured in the six components outlined in Table 5 (Barber 1983, Lee 1986, Renn & Levine 1991).

Trust relies on all six components, but a lack of compliance in one attribute can be compensated for by a surplus of goal attainment in another attribute. If objectivity or disinterestedness is impossible to accomplish, fairness of the message and faith in the good intention of the source may serve as substitutes. Competence may also be compensated by faith and empathy and vice versa. Consistency is not always essential in gaining trust, but persistent inconsistencies destroy the common expectations and role models for behavioural responses. Trust cannot evolve if people experience inconsistent responses from others in similar or even identical situations.

All public institutions have lost trust and credibility in all western countries and also in eastern Europe and beyond over the last 15 years except for the news media (Lipset & Schneider 1983). Trust and credibility losses are high for the political system and

TABLE 5 Components of trust

Components	Description
Perceived competence	Degree of technical expertise in meeting institutional mandate
Objectivity	Lack of biases in information and performance as perceived by others
Fairness	Acknowledgement and adequate representation of all relevant points of view
Consistency	Predictability of arguments and behaviour based on past experience and previous communication efforts
Sincerity	Honesty and openness
Faith	Perception of good will in performance and communication
Empathy	Caring for the victims of an accident or health-threatening release

many government agencies. Science still has a high degree of credibility, although this is much less than two decades ago. As many risk-managing agencies have been caught in the maelstrom of distrust, it is essential to revive the major elements of trust through performance and communication.

What are the most promising routes to establish trustworthiness? The first and most important recommendation is to bring institutional performance in line with the rhetorics. People lose trust in an agency or institution if promises and reality do not match. To accomplish a better match between word and deeds, honesty is a vital condition. Honesty will not automatically be rewarded, but dishonesty will certainly create negative repercussions among the media and consumers. The same effect will take place when communicators withhold relevant information or tell only one side of the story. The goals of honesty and completeness include another, often overlooked aspect. Institutions with vested interests should put their cards on the table and justify their position. Credibility is often assigned by speculating about the true motives of the source. If profits or other vested interests are obvious motives, it is better to address these issues and make clear that such interests do not automatically preclude public interest or the common good. Public utilities could, for example, make the argument that companies with a good risk reduction and control programme are more likely to attract better qualified personnel, to enhance their corporate reputation and to avoid costly litigation.

Another important method to improve trustworthiness is to be open about how decisions were made and what trade-offs were assigned between conflicting goals (such as costs versus quality). Consumers may not agree with the decision or the arguments leading to the decision, but they learn to understand the reasoning of the risk managers and the arguments that lead to the final decision. The decision-making process and the past record of the institution should be conveyed to the audience so that people can assign competence to the actors and get a better feeling of the trade-offs that had to be made in meeting the specific objective.

Perceptions and behavioural responses

Once perceptions are formed, they act as powerful agents in shaping people's responses. A major body of literature exists on how people assimilate information about hazards and transfer them into somatic or psychological effects (Aurand et al 1993). If a person feels threatened by a risk, stress and other somatic effects are likely to occur.

In order to derive an insight into the relationship between risk perception and somatic impacts, the author conducted a small psychological experiment in 1980 involving a group of 37 volunteers who were invited to a drug-testing experiment through a newspaper advertisement (Renn 1984). The participants were told the experiment was to test three different capsule coatings for possible unpleasant side-effects. It was claimed that the first capsule had a radioactive coating, the second a bacterial coating and the third an acid coating. According to the instructions given to the test subjects, all three capsules would dissolve more quickly in the stomach than conventional materials. The participants were also told that there was no health risk associated with any of the three capsules. In actual fact, the three capsules were three absolutely identical, commercially available vitamin tablets. All the subjects were then divided by random sampling into two groups of similar size (18 and 19). The first group of test persons was allowed to select one of the three capsules, and the subjects of the second group were assigned one of the three capsules by the author. Ten minutes after swallowing the capsules, the test persons had to complete a questionnaire, giving information about any discomfort and distress (e.g. stomach pains, and feeling weak or exhausted). The results of the experiment are given in Fig. 3. Although all test persons had swallowed identical capsules, the subjects of the no-choice group who had been assigned one of the capsules complained of feeling unwell more than twice as often, on average, as those subjects who had selected their capsules. This result was independent of which capsule had been chosen or had been administered in each case. In addition, the capsule that allegedly contained a radioactive coating was the most frequent cause of discomfort in both groups. The main insight of this experiment was that the strength of psychosomatic reactions depends on many conditions that may or may not be related to the actual causal agent. A sense of personal control is one among several important promoters of developing somatic symptoms as a result of a real or imagined exposure.

This finding has been substantiated by several studies on somatic reactions to nuclear accidents or radiation. Baum et al (1983) reported that persons who showed high levels of stress after the Three Mile Island accident were more convinced than others that they lacked control over their life and that they had insufficient power to protect themselves against radiation. Similarly, a survey among German men and

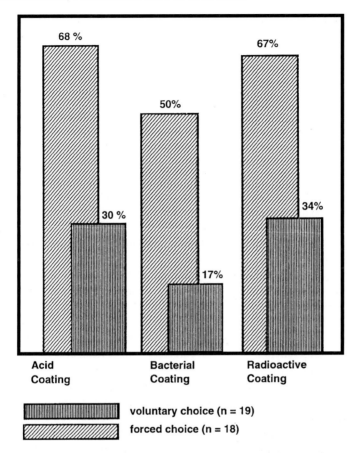

FIG. 3. Results of the drug experiment. Two groups of subjects were given conventional vitamin tablets allegedly containing either a radioactive coating, a bacterial coating or an acid coating. The first group was allowed to choose among the three capsules, the second group had no choice but was asked to take the capsule that the experiment conductor assigned to each group member. Involuntary risk exposure led to twice as many self-reported symptoms of discomfort as voluntary exposure.

women demonstrated that emotional reactions towards Chernobyl were highly associated with the belief that humans had lost control over modern technology (Hüppe & Janke 1993). Fatalism, loss of control and the extent to which people believed they could affect the amount of dose received were all relevant predictors of distress and discomfort experienced in the Russian and Ukrainian population affected by the Chernobyl accident (Rumyantseva et al 1996). Other important factors reported in this review of survey data and psychological experiments included fear of health effects for oneself and the family, followed by self-rated health and worry about social consequences of the accident, the feeling of helplessness and lack of trust in governmental bodies. These psychological problems associated with the Chernobyl accident did not decrease over time.

Distress was also a predominant feature of those people who had been resettled to other areas, in particular if the move was involuntary. Furthermore, some of the psychological factors also had an impact on the actual dose received. In conjunction with the psychological survey, people in two Russian towns underwent whole-body ^{137}Cs measurements. One of the most interesting results was that people who tend to believe that things are determined by fate were more likely to have higher dose compared to others. In this respect, psychological factors do not only influence or cause somatic reactions, but they may also control or aggravate actual exposure to a hazard.

Looking at these results, the psychological processing of information on hazards is of eminent importance in coping with psychosomatic effects. Since environmental hazards, and radiation in particular, are likely to fall in the category of 'Pandora's box' (as described above), people tend to de-emphasize probabilities and to seek additional, trustworthy information. In the case of Chernobyl, the ubiquitous nature of the hazard, the lack of sensing organs for the dangers of radiation, the worldwide attention to this accident and the helplessness of authorities in the immediate aftermath of the accident increased the feeling of being exposed to a deadly agent irrespective of dose and levels of contamination. It has been shown that psychological and social worries are largely a function of exposure and less of risk (Renn et al 1992). The more people feel exposed to a hazard and the less they feel that protective actions are available, the higher is the level of distress and discomfort even if nobody is seriously injured or harmed. This feeling is reinforced if information is ambiguous, expertise is contested and trust in local or regional authorities is eroded. Lack of understanding the nature of radiological hazards may also contribute to the stress level. A pilot study in the Gomel area in Russia showed that although 81% of the participants affirmed that they had been subjected to a medical examination due to the radiological situation after the accident, as many as 74% also reported that they did not know if they had received a dangerous dose of radiation (Rumyantseva 1996). This confusion about one's own health situation, coupled with the general problems of economic and political transition, contributed to the fact that health officials continue to report a serious increase of many somatic health effects that are clearly unrelated to the risks of radiation.

Such strong reactions to radiation hazards are not restricted to the population around Chernobyl. Particularly in Germany, people responded with many symptoms of distress and even somatic effects in the aftermath of the Chernobyl accident (Ruff 1986, Hüppe & Janke 1993). More than 50% of a German sample believed their health was threatened by radiation from Chernobyl found in food and on the ground (Hüppe & Janke 1993). More than two-thirds were confused about the information they received and complained about the ambiguities of the reports. Three-quarters of the sample were convinced that the accident demonstrated that the government will lie

TABLE 6 Psychosomatic impacts

Psychosomatic impacts	Attribute
Psychological stress	Competing information
	Reliance on information from others
	Insufficient time to cope with risk
	Loss of trust
	Loss of personal control
Suppression of health hazards	Personal interest in risk source
	Linkage between risk and highly esteemed benefit or habit (such as home)
	Apathy
	Perception of unavoidability
Amplification of health hazards	Conflicting information (better safe than sorry)
	Blame (inflicted by others)
	Exposure with stochastic effects
	Non-familiarity with hazard

to the public if a major disaster occurs. These results confirm that the three main factors, i.e. exposure, confusion and distrust, were also present in Germany as they were in Russia, Belarus or the Ukraine, and contributed to the overall stress level among the German population.

It is an interesting question to ask why environmental and particularly radiation risks are prone to induce such strong psychological impacts. Psychoanalysts have hypothesized that nature and the environment resemble sacred grounds of one's own psyche and remind people of motherhood, emotional warmth and cosmic harmony (Küchenoff 1994). If the inner-psychic harmony is distorted or threatened, a causal connection is drawn between one's own feeling and the perceived environmental degradation. Furthermore, the degradation is then rationalized as the cause for one's own health situation. Under these circumstances, all kinds of somatic symptoms are attributed to environmental hazards. Other explains for the high sensitivity of people to environmental threats include media-induced hysteria (again as part of Pandora's box), reinforcement of anxieties by social group dynamics and alienation from nature (see for a brief review Tretter 1996). Although these factors may all contribute to the magnitude and intensity of psychosomatic reactions triggered by environmental hazards, the question of why and how environmental threats trigger stress and somatic symptoms is far from being resolved. Interesting to note is that environmental threats are not only amplified, but also often attenuated (Kasperson et al 1988). Even among the people relocated from the immediate vicinity of Chernobyl, 35% of those who left voluntarily would remain in their home village if such an accident occurred again. Of those who were forced to evacuate, 50% would remain. Over-reaction to alleged dangers are part of human responses to environmental hazards as well as attenuation or even suppression of real dangers. Sometimes these responses are even mixed.

Psychosomatic reactions can hence manifest themselves in two different forms: suppression of a real health threat and amplification of perceived health risks. In both cases, psychological factors govern the human response with real improvements of clinical symptoms when exposed to placebos. On the other hand, many people feel threatened by environmental pollutants, although dose–response studies would not suggest any health effect. Table 6 provides an overview of the causes of stress, suppression of health impacts and amplification of such impacts.

The inducement of stress is likely to be linked to three major influences: real or perceived exposure to a risk agent; the perception of confusion about the risk level and appropriate reaction; and finally the perception of insufficient time to make the necessary adjustments. If one of these factors is present, people tend to respond with increased concern and worry. If all of these factors are present, combined with symbolic connotations of environmental threats and the perception of technological hubris, a response as strong as that observed in the aftermath of Chernobyl is not so surprising.

Conclusions

This list of individual and social factors that shape risk perception demonstrates that the intuitive understanding of risk is a multidimensional concept and cannot be reduced to the product of probabilities and consequences (Allen 1987). Although risk perceptions differ considerably among social and cultural groups, the multidimensionality of risk and the integration of beliefs related to risk, the cause of risk and its circumstances into a consistent belief system appear to be common characteristics of public risk perception in almost all countries in which such studies have been performed.

Risk perception studies have revealed the various elements that shape the individual and social experience of risk. First, individual and social risk experience appears to be more strongly related to exposure than to actual casualties on which most risk assessments are based. An exposure of a few people resulting in several casualties is likely to be less influential for risk perception and public response than an exposure of many people resulting in minor injuries or only few casualties. Second, the processing of risk by the media, social groups, institutions and individuals shapes the societal experience with risk and plays a crucial role in determining the overall intensity and scope of societal impacts. This finding supports the theoretical claim in the beginning of this chapter that risk reflects both real harm and social constructions. Third, individual perception is highly influenced by qualitative risk characteristics and semantic images. These images constitute tools of reducing complexity by providing easily identifiable cues for ordering new risks into one of four images:

pending danger; slow killers; cost–benefit ratios; and avocational thrill. These images are internalized through cultural and social learning. They cluster around qualitative variables that specify the context and the situation in which the risk manifests itself within each image. Although these variables allow a certain degree of abstraction with respect to perceiving and evaluating risks across different risk sources, they provide sufficient contextual specification for making the necessary semantic distinctions between negligible, serious and unacceptable risks. Abstracting the risk concept ever further and reducing it to probability and consequences violates people's intuitive feeling of what is important when making judgements about the acceptability of risks. Rather than evaluating risk with a single formula, most people use a set of multiple attributes, many of which make normative sense. The application of qualitative characteristics seems to be a universal mechanism of risk perception that has been discovered in many countries. Their specific content and relative importance depend, however, on the cultural context in which the individual is raised.

When it comes to risk responses, perception is only one influential factor among others. In this chapter I focused on three influential factors: media responses; trust in institutions; and psychosomatic reactions. They all play a major role in shaping behavioural responses to risk and structuring risk debates. In a social environment in which personal experience is largely constructed by second-hand information, trust is an essential prerequisite for communication and social co-ordination. Trust can easily be destroyed by non-predictable or non-avoidable disasters; at the same time it can easily be exploited by referring to random events as explanations or excuses for risk management errors or hubris. As both processes occur simultaneously, trust is constantly at stake in institutional responses to risk. One way to cope with this problem is to develop an organizational style that either leads to high reliability performance or to immunization against public scrutiny. In a situation where people feel threatened by a risk source, they are likely to develop a feeling of unease and even clinical symptoms. The somatic system is closely linked to psychological influences.

How can risk perception be improved by means of risk communication? Careful management, openness to public demands and continuous efforts to communicate are important conditions for successful risk communication. Gaining trust-worthiness and competence depend primarily on a good performance record. Is the performance good enough to justify public trust? Are mechanisms in place that help to discern the needs and requests of stakeholders and the general public? Is a two-way communication programme implemented? Is the communication honest, clear, comprehensive and timely?

If these questions can be positively answered, the designing of communication can be optimized. The major guideline here is to tailor communication according to the needs of the targeted audience and not to the needs of the information source. Providing information that people request is always more effective than providing answers to questions that nobody has asked. By carefully reviewing in-house performance, by tailoring the content of the communication to the needs of the final receivers, and by adjusting the messages to the values and concerns of the audience, risk communication can convey a basic understanding for the choices and constraints of risk management and thus create the foundations for a trustworthy relationship between the communicator and the audience. Although many receivers of risk information may not agree with the actual decisions institutions have made in setting priorities or selecting management options, they may realize that these decisions are results of open discussions and the assignment of painful trade-offs.

References

Adams WC 1986 Whose lives count?: TV coverage of natural disasters. Communication 36:113–122

Allen FW 1987 Towards a holistic appreciation of risk: the challenge for communicators and policy-makers. Science Technol Hum Values 12:138–143

Aurand K, Hazard B, Tretter F 1993 Umweltbelastungen und Ängste. Westdeutscher Verlag, Opladen

Barber B 1983 The logic and limits of trust. Rutgers University Press, New Brunswick, NJ

Baum A, Gatchel RJ, Scheaffer MA 1983 Emotional, behavioral and physiological effects of stress at Three Mile Island. J Consult Psychol 51:565–572

Chaiken S, Stangor C 1987 Attitudes and attitude change. Annu Rev Psychol 38:575–630

Clarke L 1989 Acceptable risk?: making decisions in a toxic environment. University of California Press, Berkeley, CA

Coombs B, Slovic P 1979 Newspaper coverage of causes of death. Journalism Quart 56:837–849

Covello VT 1983 The perception of technological risks: a literature review. Technol Forecast & Soc Change 23:285–297

Dunwoody S 1992 The media and public perception of risk: how journalists frame risk stories. In: DW Bromley (ed) The social response to environmental risk: policy formulation in an age of uncertainty. Kluwer, Dordrecht, p 236–263

Festinger L 1957 A theory of cognitive dissonance. Stanford University Press, Stanford, CA

Gould LC, Gardner GT, DeLuca DR et al 1988 Perceptions of technological risks and benefits. Russel Sage Foundation, New York

Hüppe M, Janke W 1993 Empirische Befunde zur Wirkung vom Umweltkatastrophen auf das Erleben und die Stressverarbeitung von Männern und Frauen unterschiedlichen Alters. In: Aurand K, Hazaer B, Tretter F (eds) Umweltbelastungen und Ängste. Westdeutscher Verlag, Opladen, p 133–144

Kahneman D, Tversky A 1979 Prospect theory: an analysis of decision under risk. Econometrica 47:263–291

Kasperson RE, Kasperson JX 1983 Determining the acceptability of risk: ethical and policy issues. In: Rogers JT, Bates DV (eds) Assessment and perception of risk to human health. Conference Proceedings of the conference on Assessment and perception of risk to human health, Sept 1982, Ottawa, Royal Society of Canada, p 135–155

Kasperson RE, Renn O, Slovic P et al 1988 The social amplification of risk: a conceptual framework. Risk Analysis 8:177–187

Küchenhoff C 1994 Umwelt-Psychosomatik. In: Beyer A, Eis D (eds) Praktische Umweltmedizin. Springer-Verlag, Berlin

Lee TR 1981 The public perception of risk and the question of irrationality. In: The Royal Society of Great Britain (ed) Risk perception, vol 376. The Royal Society, London, p 5–16

Lee TR 1986 Effective communication of information about chemical hazards. Sci Total Environ 51:49–183

Lichtenberg J, MacLean D 1988 The role of the media in risk communication. In: Jungermann H, Kasperson RE, Wiedemann PM (eds) Risk communication. Nuclear Research Center, Jülich, p 33–48

Lipset SM, Schneider W 1983 The confidence gap, business, labor, and government in the public mind. The Free Press, New York

Lopes LL 1983 Some thoughts on the psychological concept of risk. J Exp Psychol Hum Percept Perform 9:137–144

Luce RD, Weber EU 1986 An axiomatic theory of conjoint expected risk. J Math Psychol 30:188–205

Luhmann N 1986 kologische Kommunikation. Westdeutscher Verlag, Opladen

Luhmann N 1990 Technology, environment and social risk: a systems perspective. Indust Crisis Quart 4:223–231

Machlis GE, Rosa EA 1990 Desired risk: broadening the social amplification of risk framework. Risk Analysis 10:161–168

McCombs MD, Shaw DL 1972 The agenda-setting function of mass media. Public Op Q 36:176–182

NRC 1983 Risk assessment in the federal government: managing the process. National Research Council, committee on the institutional means for assessment of risks to the public health. National Acad Press, Washington DC

Otway H, Thomas K 1982 Reflections on risk perception and policy. Risk Analysis 2:69–82

Peltu M 1985 The role of communications media. In: Otway H, Peltu M (eds) Regulating industrial risks. Butterworth, London, p 128–148

Peltu M 1988 Media reporting of risk information: uncertainties and the future. In: Jungermann H, Kasperson RE, Wiedemann PM (eds) Risk communication. Nuclear Research Centre, Jülich, p 11–31

Peters HP 1984 Entstehung Verarbeitung und Verbreitung von Wissenschaftsnachrichten am Beispiel von 20 Forschungseinrichtungen. Nuclear Research Center, Jülich

Peters HP 1991 Durch Risikokommunikation zur Technikakzeptanz? Die Konstruktion von Risiko'wirklichkeiten' durch Experten Gegenexperten und ffentlichkeit. In: Krüger J, Ruß-Mohl S (eds) Risikokommunikation: Technikakzeptanz, Medien und Kommunikationsrisiken. Edition Sigma, Berlin, p 11–16

Petty RE, Cacioppo E 1986 The elaboration likelihood model of persuasion. Adv Exp Soc Psychol 19:123–205

Pollatsek A, Tversky A 1970 A theory of risk. J Math Psychol 7:540–553

Raymond CA 1985 Risk in the press: conflicting journalistic ideologies. In: D Nelkin (ed) The language of risk: conflicting perspectives on occupational health. Books on Demand, Ann Arbor, MI, p 97–133

Renn O 1984 Risikowahrnehmung der Kernenergie. Campus, Frankfurt

Renn O 1986 Akzeptanzforschung: Technik in der gesellschaftlichen Auseinander-setzung. Chem unserer Zeit 2:44–52

Renn O 1989 Risk communication in the community: European lessons from the Seveso directive. J Air Pollut Control Assoc 40:1301–1308

Renn O 1990a Risk perception and risk management: a review. I. Risk Abstr 7:1–9

Renn O 1990b Risk perception and risk management: a review. II. Risk Abstr 7:1–9

Renn O 1992 Concepts of risk: a classification. In: Krimsky S, Golding D (eds) Social theories of risk. Praeger, Westport, CT, p 53–79

Renn O, Levine D 1991 Trust and credibility in risk communication. In: Kasperson RE, Stallen PJ (eds) Communicating risk to the public: international perspectives. Kluwer, Dordrecht, p 175–218

Renn O, Burns W, Kasperson RE, Kasperson JX, Slovic P 1992 The social amplification of risk: theoretical foundations and empirical application. Soc Iss 48:137–160

Ross LD 1977 The intuitive psychologist and his shortcomings: distortions in the attribution process. In: Berkowitz L(ed) Advances in experimental social psychology, vol 10. Academic Press, London, p 173–220

Rubin DM 1987 How the news media reported on Three Mile Island and Chernobyl. Communication 37:42–57

Ruff FM 1986 Psychische Folgen von Reaktorunfällen-Langzeitstress nach der Reaktorkatastrophe von Three Mile Island (Harrisburg). Verhaltenstherapie und psychosoziale Praxis 18:498–508

Rumyanseva GM, Drottz-Sjöberg B-M, Allen PT et al 1996 The influence of social and psychological factors in the management of contaminated territories. In: The radiological consequences of the Chernobyl accident. The European Commission and the Belarus, Russian and Ukrainian ministries on Chernobyl affairs, emergency situations and health (eds) Report EUR 16544 EN, European Commission, Brussels

Short JF 1984 The social fabric of risk: toward the social transformation of risk analysis. Am Sociol Rev 9:711–725

Short JF 1989 On defining describing and explaining elephants (and reactions to them): hazards disasters and risk analysis. Mass Emerg Disasters 7:397–418

Slovic P 1987 Perception of risk. Science 236:280–285

Slovic P, Fischhoff B, Lichtenstein S 1981 Perceived risk: psychological factors and social implications. In: The Royal Society (ed) Proceedings of the Royal Society A376. The Royal Society, London, p 17–34

Sood R, Stockdale G, Rogers EM 1987 How the news media operate in natural disasters. Communication 37:27–41

Thomas K, Maurer D, Fishbein M, Otway HJ, Hinkle R, Simpson DA 1980 Comparative study of public beliefs about five energy systems. International Institute for Applied Systems Analysis Report 80–15, IIASA, Laxenburg, Austria

Tretter F 1996 Umwelt und Psyche. In: Umweltministerium und Ministerium für Arbeit, Gesundheit und Sozialordnung (eds) Macht uns die Umwelt Krank? Proceedings of the Health and Environmental Congress, Dec 6 1995 in Stuttgart. Environmental Ministry, Karlsruhe 81–100

Vlek CAJ, Stallen PJ 1981 Judging risks and benefits in the small and in the large. Org Behav Hum Perform 28:235–271

Wilkins L, Patterson P 1987 Risk analysis and the construction of news. Communication 37:80–92

DISCUSSION

Aarkrog: You mentioned that the credibility of scientific institutions has decreased over the last 15 years, whereas the media has not lost any credibility. Are these two observations related?

Renn: Yes. The credibilities of the media and the scientific institutions are to a large extent inversely related. It's almost like a homeostatic situation: there is a certain amount of credibility that needs to be assigned to someone, and one community's loss is another's gain. For example, in Germany after the Chernobyl accident the credibility of some of the established research organizations decreased, whereas the credibility of ecologically oriented research organizations and the media increased. In both western Europe and the USA, the total amount of credibility towards the sciences has decreased.

Roed: I have the opposite impression of the situation during the Chernobyl accident. Before the accident the Danish press consulted the environmentalists, and not the experts, but after the accident they put their questions to the experts, and there seemed to be no reports from those who were not experts. This resulted in the experts having a high credibility in this situation.

Renn: This may be true for Denmark, but the empirical data show a clear decline in perceived trustworthiness for the established research organizations and an increase for ecologically oriented institutions. However, there are other cases of the kind that you mentioned. Immediately after the Brent Spar incident, Greenpeace had a high credibility. However, once Greenpeace won the case, the situation changed dramatically because Greenpeace was perceived as a big and powerful player. Good intentions were not enough any more. The public then questioned the science and the decision-making structure. Counter-forces in society are often forgiven for perceived incompetence because they raise a lot of empathy, but once they become powerful agents, they are subjected to the same degree of scrutiny as established forces.

Whicker: When I first started dealing with the concept of uncertainty I realized that it was a way of being honest with everything. Yet, when I tell the lay person that our models are only reliable to within a factor of 10, for example, they get the impression that the science is bad. Could you comment on this problem?

Renn: This is an important observation and there is no easy answer because it may be a no-win situation. If you don't talk about uncertainty, when people face a collective risk, an informed person in the audience will pick you up on it and accuse you of lying or playing down the point. This situation is almost impossible to rescue because if the rest of the audience doesn't understand the point they think you are being caught in the middle of a manipulation attempt. On the other hand, if you inform the audience about all the uncertainties and tell them, for example, that in a linear dose–response relationship even a very small dose has a very small probability of inducing cancer, people will feel that the situation is unacceptable because any person may eventually be affected. I feel that informing the public about uncertainties, being honest and showing a sense of respect for the phenomenon that you're dealing with is more convincing than telling them that you are more certain about your research results than you actually are. People prefer certainty. They have been trained in schools that science can give definite answers to all factual questions, which of course is not true, so you are operating against a powerful prejudice. But, in the long run, an honest approach conveys a degree of modesty in the sense that we don't know everything and that we like to empower people to make their own decision. This brings up the issue of control. We can state what we know, but what is done with that knowledge is often a decision of lifestyle or politics, i.e. we can tell an individual what we as persons would do in their position but it's up to that individual to make his or her own decision.

Howard: The willingness to discuss uncertainty and rationale behind decision making often conflicts with what is required from us, by either the public or the media, because they want us to generalize.

Renn: The media play an important role because direct experience has only a limited impact when we talk about radiation. The lay public has no other choice but to believe the media. This is not only true for radiation but also, for example, if I watch television and I see a reporter in Bosnia telling me about the situation there I don't know whether what they are saying is true or not. It is up to me to trust them. Turning back to risks, the media have an interest in the social experience of risk — that is, how people perceive and respond to risk — and not really in the risk numbers. In addition, insights from the study of social processing of risk have shown us that exposure is always more important than damage. When dealing with the media, it is advisable to acknowledge that they are interested in reporting all angles of a case rather than a specific point of view. One should also be aware that media coverage is a function of political exposure, of political conflict and anticipated concern of the public. It is possible to deliver uncertainty information within the framework of these journalistic features. However, I suggest that you do not compromise your messages just to please the media. In the long run, if you overextend your scientific competence into areas in which you're not competent and someone finds out about it, it's difficult for you to regain your credibility.

Goldman: One disturbing trend is that the total immersion of society in technology seems, in my opinion, to be based on public perception. This is evolving into a situation in which the scientists are being blamed for everything. From the public's point of view, most of the things that we do either don't work or create problems, which is generating a somewhat anti-technology attitude. The problem is exacerbated by the public's willingness to believe anecdotal reports, no matter how irrational they are, rather than listen to a scientist. Could you comment on this?

Renn: Perception of science follows the movement of a pendulum. In the 1950s and 1960s science was often perceived as a new religion. This perception has largely vanished, and to some extent the pendulum has swung the other way. However, there is still a minority of people who feel that science has introduced all the technological, environmental and economic problems that we suffer from. The percentage of people who are truly anti-science is less than 5% in western countries. The people who are completely pro-science is about 10%. The remaining portion of the public is ambiguous and is becoming more sceptical about the promises of science and technology to society. If ambiguity arises, credibility becomes the major issue because ambiguity demands to know both sides of the story. The media will always present both sides, but one side is usually more convincing. Scepticism towards science and technology is not only found in most western countries. This is also true in most eastern countries. Credibility towards science has been reported as rather low in most surveys around the Chernobyl area.

Streffer: I would like you to comment on two points. First, do you have any information about subpopulations, especially with respect to education? Although illiteracy is increasing in Germany, it's probably fair to say that education has never been of such a high standard as it is today: about 40% of the population go to high school and about 25% go to university. I was therefore disappointed that you seemed to down-play the role of perceived competence as a component of trust. I would expect that if the level of education is increasing that competence should be more acknowledged.

Second, I have the impression from my experiences of the Chernobyl accident that if people are directly involved, then their awareness increases and competence becomes more important. I had to give several talks during the first few weeks after the accident and the lecture rooms were always full. People were eager to obtain any kind of information, and they recognized the people who wanted to disturb the lecture and were not interested in the information. However, after a few months the situation and danger had smoothed down, and the lecture rooms became emptier and the discussions became increasingly more difficult and irrational. People who claimed unreasonable things got more and more resonance.

Renn: Firstly, literacy and competence of the public has improved in most countries. One of the big myths is that, with increased technical literacy, the attitude towards either technology or science will become more positive. We are talking here about basic level of literacy. What you may feel somebody needs to know about radiology will apply to less than 1% of the population. Yet those people may still have a fair knowledge of everything. There are so many different fields today that no one has the ability or the time to know more than the simple basics of a subject. Taking the basic knowledge as a predictor for attitudes has been proven wrong in many surveys. The correlation between, for example, knowledge about either nuclear energy or radionuclides and one's attitudes towards nuclear power is close to zero. So, it is not knowledge that counts in the interaction between a scientist and a member of the public, but perceived competence. If people listen to arguments about nuclear energy, they don't have the knowledge to distinguish between who is right or wrong. Therefore, attributing competence is based on other criteria, such as sympathy and perceived (hidden) interests.

Your second point is, in a sense, related to this. As soon as one obtains some level of competence through direct experience, people automatically switch to the central route of information processing and they want to hear arguments. If they don't hear good arguments, they feel that there's not much competence behind the arguments given to them. If direct experience is missing, people shift towards the peripheral route and the symbolic cues become more important. In this case it's not the quality of the argument that convinces, it's the quality of the presentation or the package.

Goldman: How do you explain the increased credibility for an entertainer to be involved with sensitive issues and have an enormous following? One frequently sees debates where technical experts are up against film stars, and the film stars win. They are much more articulate and usually better looking, but I don't understand why this makes them more credible.

Renn: A film star has a degree of openness to public demands, and they act personally and authentically, even though their scientific competence is regarded as low. They usually have a high level of empathy for those involved in the same situation and they often highlight the impacts on children, which in turn guarantees the public sympathy. A scientist who presents data and figures in such an emotional case is almost bound to lose. Therefore, it is important to put the data into context and show a large degree of empathy with potential victims.

Frissel: I am from The Netherlands, which is protected by dykes. The probability that a dyke will collapse is 1 : 3000, but if it does there will be hundreds of thousands of casualties. This carries a higher risk compared to the risks involved with nuclear energy and it is more dangerous, yet no one worries about the dykes collapsing. Why is this?

Renn: This is a common pattern. Dams and dykes are not put into the impending danger category, they are put in the category of natural hazards. Natural hazards are viewed in a totally different way. For example, people always come back to an area that has been flooded, even though they know there is still a high probability that the area will experience floods again. There are two reasons for this: first, they have the impression that a natural disaster is 'an act of God' and there is no one to blame; and second, the probabilities are perceived differently, i.e. 1 : 3000 is not seen as something that can happen tomorrow, but that if the region has recently been flooded it will take another 3000 years before it is flooded again. Technological hazards, however, are perceived as something that may happen again, even directly after an accident. Purely from a statistical point of view, this doesn't make sense. However, we need to bear in mind that the familiarity which people have of natural hazards makes it easier for them to accept a low probability risk; whereas such a familiarity is lacking in the case of technological hazards, for which they don't have an immediate mental image.

Lake: Do large releases of radionuclides cause damage to mental health through paranoia, for example?

Renn: There is a debate as to whether clinical evidence on psychosis induced by radiophobia actually exists. I am cautious of this hypothesis because most phobic responses, specifically in western Europe, are temporary phenomena. After the Chernobyl accident there were reports of many responses that were totally out of proportion compared to the actual threat. However, most of the symptoms were not sustained over a long period of time, which would have suggested psychotic phobias. There is, however, a tendency of increasing numbers of people to feel affected by environmental hazards or radiation. As I pointed out, a causal connection to a physical agent is often difficult to draw or even clearly absent. In such cases, people feel threatened by environmental factors for a variety of reasons and show somatic reactions as a result of these perceptions.

Paretzke: There were two newspaper reports in Bavaria in the summer of 1986 that described medical doctors shooting their families and themselves because they felt that they had failed to protect them from the contamination. Therefore, these psychotic responses to perceived risks are real health hazards.

Streffer: For clarification I would like to say that, from the clinical point of view, there are no data that irradiation causes such psychotic effects directly.

Cigna: Can you give us some guidelines on how to deal with the public's perception of risk?

Renn: There are two important aspects, which I have mentioned already.

First, it is important to give people the impression that what you are working on is fascinating but that it still remains a miracle or mystery. The more you uncover the mystery, the more you frighten people, which is just the opposite of what you might expect. It is important to state that you share a great respect for the natural forces that are at work in a nuclear reactor. The worst you can do is convey over-confidence. The Chernobyl accident should never have happened, not because the technology involved was at fault, but because it was triggered by the over-confidence of the personnel, who believed they could master any dangerous situation.

Second, you must be authentic about your own motives and concerns. Authenticity is something that people value because nowadays they are bombarded with second-hand information and they frequently experience that they are being cheated. They must realize that you are a human being and that you empathize with them. If you can convey to them that you share their concerns, worries and anxieties, they can relate to you and you gain credibility. However, these feelings need to be true!

Final discussion

Voigt: I would like to ask Marvin Goldman to comment on the development of cataracts in eye lenses.

Goldman: Radiation can induce cataracts in eyes, which are particularly sensitive to exposure to neutrons. We obtained most of this information from the early cyclotron workers who were exposed to rather large doses. The evidence suggests that for low linear energy transfer radiation, there is a threshold for this condition (ICRP 1984). It is not a stochastic process, in that a certain amount of injury to the lens tissue must occur before these cataracts become manifest. There is one report of a possible increase in cataracts in some of the Chernobyl liquidators, although the dosimetry is still not complete. It doesn't seem to be dependent on sex or age, although the number of cases is small. The development of a cataract is not a sensitive indicator, it takes a large dose in the order of 0.6 Gy, and there is also a long latency period of about five years.

Paretzke: If a person has a suspected acute external exposure of 0.2 Gy which method would you recommend for analysing this person a year later?

Goldman: A quick analysis could be done with the micronucleus test. I would also do a T lymphocyte count if I wanted to confirm that they had received an acute dose, because they would be decreased in number. The standard chromosome aberration analysis, i.e. of rings and dicentrics, could also be done rapidly. I would only do the more sophisticated fluorescence *in situ* hybridization (FISH) technique after I had established that the received dose was around 0.2 Gy.

Paretzke: I would like to ask the same question to Manfred Bauchinger.

Bauchinger: A conventional dicentric analysis would be sufficient after one year. I would not recommend the FISH technique because it's expensive and at that low dose level, for statistical reasons, one would need to score about 4000 cells. Although this could be achieved in one day, because it's 10 times quicker to score than by conventional staining, for an examination of a large group of exposed persons, automatic scoring would be highly desirable.

Goldman: What would be useful to have on the record is some sort of a triage so that specific procedures are followed when the doses are large, intermediate and small. As far as I know, there isn't a universal agreement on how to do this.

Paretzke: So what would you recommend should be done if a large group of people received a suspected dose of 1 Gy?

Goldman: If the dose was 1 Gy, one would immediately recognize those people who are sensitive because they will develop symptoms of radiation sickness, i.e. nausea, vomiting and diarrhoea. These people would require immediate clinical care. The classical, simple haematological parameters (which are not recommended for low dose exposure) would be relatively reliable for this dose. If I was involved in a legal case, in which it was essential that I documented the exposure in detail irrespective of the cost, then I would do the FISH analysis because this would reduce the uncertainty to the minimum.

Bauchinger: It would also be necessary to do cumulated blood cell counts, and particularly T lymphocyte counts. I would recommend a conventional chromosome analysis and, for a rapid screening procedure, the micronucleus assay may also be used; however, one should do this latter test as a cell cycle-controlled approach using the cytochalasin B technique. The FISH technique with a centromere probe provides the information on the contents of the micronuclei, i.e. whether only acentric fragments or complete chromosomes are present. It would not be necessary to score large numbers of cells for chromosome analysis immediately after a radiation accident. Scoring of 50–100 cells does not provide meaningful information about the dose distribution but it can be sufficient for a rapid selection of radiation victims requiring preventive medical treatment.

Voigt: These procedures would be restricted to a small number of people because they are too expensive and time consuming. What would you recommend for the dose reconstruction of larger population groups?

Bauchinger: They are not too expensive but there are logistic problems if larger populations have been exposed. However, as exemplified for the Chernobyl and Goiania radiation accidents, about 100 and 200 victims, respectively, could be examined during the first days and weeks after the accident. It is remarkable that the first information on individual doses was achieved from biological dosimetry based on chromosome aberrations and blood cell counts. There is no doubt about the importance of physical dose measurements; however, for an individual diagnostic evaluation or an assessment of the homogeneity of exposure with respect to an ultimate decision for a bone marrow transplantation, a biological dose estimation is mandatory.

Goldman: But in terms of a large population, if your job was to convince the population that the dose was small, then the conventional cytogenetic test for 100 people or so would be inadequate. You would probably have, at the same time, enough environmental dose reconstruction to support your results. I would like to stress that the first thing I would do is obtain the physical data. You need to know if there's a reason to expect the absorbed doses to be high.

Streffer: I agree with what Marvin Goldman and Manfred Bauchinger have said but I would also like to point out that from biological dosimetry one can obtain information not only about the dose exposure but also about the variations in radiosensitivity of the individuals.

Paretzke: Is there any indication that people who are more sensitive to high therapeutic doses of radiation are also more likely to develop cancer from low dose irradiation?

Streffer: We don't yet have these data for ionizing irradiation. However, we have had clinical experiences in radiotherapy where people are sensitive to ionizing irradiation, in that they develop side-effects in normal tissues. If we do cytogenetic tests on these people, we observe an increased frequency of chromosomal aberrations. We have observed this in ataxia telangiectasia patients and in people who suffer from Fanconi's anaemia. At the moment, we can only assume that these people are more likely to develop cancer. We know that they have a higher risk of developing spontaneous cancer but we don't know whether this is also true for ionizing radiation.

Goldman: It's important to stress that a good biological indicator does not give any indication of that individual's subsequent cancer risk. We have many clues, but no hard data. In the case of Fanconi's anaemia, we know that there is a predisposition to leukaemia because of the abnormal way in which the stem cells are constructed. There are those who think that we all have a unique soft spot in our genome but we don't have any proof of this.

Streffer: I agree in principle but we need to identify the people who require cancer screening, so that we may be able to detect cancers at an early stage.

Bauchinger: I agree that the ultimate goal is to identify radiosensitive people but, because of the time pressures involved in the screening of hundreds of people, it is unlikely that we will be able to do this.

Goldman: There is much work to be done, but we have to be realistic and optimistic about these approaches.

Reference

ICRP 1984 Non-stochastic effects of ionizing radiation International Commission on Radiation Protection publication 41. Pergamon, Oxford

Summary

Herwig G. Paretzke

GSF, Institut für Strahlenschutz, Imgolstädter Landstrasse 1, 857 64 Neuherberg, Germany

During this symposium on the health impacts of large releases of radionuclides we have heard many interesting presentations and we have had equally interesting discussions. It was extremely valuable to have sufficient time to discuss the many important points raised in each presentation. It has become clear that radioactivity in the environment is an important tool for general scientific research as well as an object of research.

Radioactive isotopes emit ionizing irradiation, which can disturb biological systems. Only after a challenging disturbance is it possible to study the dynamic responses, actions or repair processes of such systems. Over the past decades, insight into cellular processes, carcinogenesis and other processes determining human life has been gained by the use of ionizing radiation. However, we have also had to learn of many detrimental effects of radiation on human life. Radionuclides in the environment have an important property in that they can be used as a moving clock, with a label indicating their origin in time and space. If the ratio of isotopes in a quantity of water, for example, at the time of emission is known, because of the rules of radioactive decay, it is often possible to calculate the 'age', i.e. the transport time from a source, of a particular sample of water, and from where it could have come. Similar considerations apply in atmospheric transport measurements as well as in transport within the food-chain.

Radioisotope labelling is also used as a sensitive atom detection method in other scientific studies. By neutron activation and fission fragment analysis it is possible to determine how many plutonium atoms are exhaled by an individual in a few litres of air. At this symposium we dealt with the behaviour of radionuclides in the environment, their transfer to humans and their effects on several aspects of human health. We looked at the various exposure pathways and transition probabilities involved in these processes, radiation action mechanisms, how to measure doses retrospectively by both physical and biological methods, and reasons for the widely observed radiation hysteria in politics, in the media and in some members of the public. We heard important arguments concerning why our daily lives in radiation sciences are affected by the public's perception of risk, which is presently seriously distorted. I sometimes wonder how much time scientists working in this challenging, interdisciplinary field should actually devote to trying to solve these types of psychosomatic problems. Precious research time will be needed to solve the many important questions left open after 10 years of intensified research in radioecology and radiation biology in, for example, the scientific follow-up after the Chernobyl reactor accident. Among these are:

(1) the quantification of the transport of pollutants in the atmosphere and in water bodies;
(2) the movement of deposited pollutants through agricultural, semi-natural, natural and urban environments;
(3) the quantification of behaviours of members of the public;
(4) the impact of radiation exposures at low total doses and at a chronic, low dose rate on human health; and
(5) improvements in our ability to estimate in a quick and reliable way such exposures retrospectively for large population groups.

However, I believe that all participants of this symposium will agree with the statement that the presentations at this meeting provided us with an excellent summary of the achievements that have been made and that the subsequent discussions indicated many possible ways of addressing the remaining questions.

Index of contributors

Non-participating co-authors are indicated by asterisks. Entries in bold type indicate papers; other entries refer to discussion contributions.

Indexes compiled by Liza Weinkove

Subject index

Other Ciba Foundation Symposia:

No. 202 **Evolution of hydrothermal ecosystems on Earth (and Mars?)**
Chairman: Malcolm R. Walter
1996 ISBN 0 471 96509 X

No. 206 **The rising trends in asthma**
Chairman: Stephen T. Holgate
1997 ISBN 0 471 97012 3

No. 207 **Antibiotic resistance: origins, evolution, selection and spread**
Chairman: Stuart Levy
1997 ISBN 0 471 97105 7